SLIMFASTING—

The Quick "Pounds Off"
Way to Youthful Slimness

Carlson Wade

Foreword by William S. Keezer, M.D.

Parker Publishing Company, Inc.

West Nyack, New York

Library of Congress Cataloging in Publication Data

Wade, Carlson.
    Slimfasting.

    Includes index.
    1. Fasting. 2. Reducing diets. 3. Food,
Natural. I. Title.
RM226.5.W3   613.2'5   77-24264
ISBN 0-13-813022-1

Printed in the United States of America

Foreword by a Doctor of Medicine

Slimfasting is the best guide to weight reduction to be published thus far. Carlson Wade, an outstanding and highly respected nutrition reporter, makes available to the public, for the first time, the entire program of fasting as a means of permanent weight loss.

Complete in this one volume, Carlson Wade has gathered the secrets of swift weight loss from long-forgotten scrolls, archives, forbidden records, modern medical-scientific revelations. He has updated these little-known health and rejuvenation secrets. He presents them in an easy-to-read outlined form for the modern reader.

Now you can tap the gold mine of weight reduction and health knowledge as drawn from hundreds of civilizations throughout tens of hundreds of centuries from all parts of the ancient and modern world.

Slimfasting, as it is called, is a dynamic new, all-natural solution to the problem of overweight. Carlson Wade, world famous medical researcher and author, shows you how to keep on eating most of your favorite foods and still take off inch after inch, pound after pound.

Thanks to Slimfasting, you can forget about hard dieting. No endless glasses of water. No costly and oft-dangerous diet pills. No clumsy calorie calculating. No artificial sweeteners. No starvation.

Instead, Carlson Wade shows you how to enjoy luscious meats, creamy dairy foods, chewy breads, delicious eggs, succulent fruits and vegetables, hearty soups, filling casseroles, sweet puddings and desserts—*and still lose weight swiftly and permanently.*

No other available diet is so effective as Carlson Wade's Slimfasting. It melts inches and pounds right before your very eyes. Carlson Wade has wisely included a delicious variety of different programs to suit every need, circumstance, taste, condition. He shows you how to *simultaneously* revitalize your body while the pounds melt away. He shows you how to firm up your body, your skin, boost your health, supercharge your energy factors, all during Slimfasting.

Carlson Wade's Slimfasting is successful because it does not blame the overeater. Instead, it goes to the root-cause of overeating and shows how you can easily correct it. Carlson Wade offers a *solution* to the problem of overeating through Slimfasting.

For a reducing program to be effective, it must satisfy your appetite, digestion, emotions and health needs. Of all the diets available, only Carlson Wade's Slimfasting fulfills all of these important needs.

Some of the program's unique features that are custom-made for almost any circumstance include:

- One-day, three-day, weekend Slimfasting programs.
- A raw juice fast shrinks stubborn bulges.
- Create internal combustion and slim down fat cells with certain everyday foods.
- Fill up on fiber and boost health while you lose weight.
- Official U.S. Government calorie charts and recommendations for weight control.
- Herbs and spices put a natural control on your appetite.
- Behavior therapy tips and tricks to retrain your eating habits.
- A salt-free Slimfasting program to shrink inches and wash out pounds. Special chart listing sodium-salt content of most foods.
- A set of 15 different Slimfasting programs to satisfy almost any need and taste. Easy 10-step planning program.
- How to use Slimfasting to rejuvenate your skin and shape-up your body.
- Slimfasting questions and answers.
- And many, many more.

Anyone who has tried to lose weight knows that the road is difficult. Now Carlson Wade has supplied solutions to all weight problems. He gets to the root-cause of overweight. He shows you how to correct the cause quickly. Then you watch stubborn fat slough right out of your body. Slimfasting shows you how to lose overweight *with* food and not without it!

Does this sound too easy? It is easy! Carlson Wade has made it so simple that almost anyone with any kind of weight problem will be able to solve it through Slimfasting. He takes you by the hand, shows you how to plan for Slimfasting, how to begin, how to continue, how to go off the program after losing your desired overweight. He includes hundreds of little known one-minute tricks to help you keep slim forever.

You'll be delighted with the results of this successful new guide to the simple, quick, effective way to be permanently slim.

Is today the day you want to melt away unwanted inches and pounds? Then begin reading the first chapter. It will change your weight. It will rejuvenate your total body and mind!

William S. Keezer, M.D.

Other Books by the Author

Helping Your Health with Enzymes
Magic Minerals: Key to Better Health
The Natural Way to Health Through Controlled Fasting
Carlson Wade's Gourmet Health Foods Cookbook
Natural and Folk Remedies
The Natural Laws of Healthful Living
Health Tonics, Elixirs and Potions for the
 Look and Feel of Youth
Natural Hormones: The Secret of Youthful Health
Health Secrets from the Orient
Magic Enzymes: Key to Youth and Health
The Miracle of Organic Vitamins for Better Health
Miracle Protein: Secret of Natural Cell-Tissue Rejuvenation
All-Natural Pain Relievers
How to Achieve Fast, Permanent Weight Loss with the
 New Enzyme-Catalyst Diet
Brand Name Handbook of Protein, Calories and Carbohydrates

What This Book Will Do for You

This book will fulfill your dreams of losing weight and keeping it off, *forever.*

Slimfasting—a long-forgotten, ancient secret of swift weight loss—is now updated and presented in a step-by-step method.

Slimfasting takes you by the hand, shows you how to *free yourself forever* from "stubborn pounds," "thick" bulges, and "lumpy" inches. This book gives you all the easy-to-follow programs you need to release and "wash out" unwanted pounds from any and all parts of your body. This book is your complete guide to a new slender shape and healthy body that will radiate the joys of youthful slimness from head to toe.

Slimfasting, as fully outlined in this book, was created for millions of "problem" overweights such as yourself. You distrust reducing drugs because of risky reactions. You are disappointed in rigorous exercises that are tiring but not too slimming. You dislike the inconvenience of impersonal group "fatty clubs."

Instead, you want an all-natural and effective slimming program to follow at home. You are searching for a simple but effective "no-fault" pound-losing program that will give you swift, permanent weight loss. That is why this book was written. To help you lose weight without drugs, without strenuous exercise, without hunger pangs! To help you conquer fat forever! To help you enjoy permanent slimness for your entire lifespan!

The key to Slimfasting's success is in its "magic ingredient." It gets to the cause of overweight. It works to loosen up accumulated "fat blocks" and then wash them out of your system. Once your vital organs are liberated from these "fat congestions," your body's weight-burning powers are released to melt away pounds and inches. Slimfasting reshapes your inside and then rejuvenates your outside. Simultaneously, as weight is lost, health is restored—rebuilt so that you emerge looking and feeling youthful and refreshingly energetic.

This book gives you a completely new approach to weight loss.

It shows you how to shed stubborn weight while enjoying favorite beverages, fruits, vegetables, casseroles, meats, and even delicious desserts.

Slimfasting shows you how to eliminate hunger pangs, how to control your appetite, how to chew and lose weight, how to use behavior therapy, how to erase so-called "middle-age spread."

There is a Slimfasting program to satisfy every taste and personal need. Get to the root of your overweight by slimming down your "fat cells" with a variety of different Slimfasting programs. Try it one day, one week, one month or longer, and watch pounds roll away.

Troubled with hunger pangs? This book gives you over 100 Slimfasting tricks and tips. They soothe your runaway appetite and satisfy your stomach so that you feel comfortably "filled up" as you slim down.

Are you an emotionally upset compulsive eater? This book describes ready-to-use "behavior therapy" to retrain your "mind's eye" so that "thought control" becomes "weight control."

Is your overweight caused by mischievous glands and imbalanced hormones? This book shows you how to adjust your "biological clocks" so your glands send forth fat-melting hormones. They help you lose weight while you sleep!

These and many, many more Slimfasting programs are fully described. All are ready for you to use at once. They help solve just about any stubborn weight problem.

No medicines. No exercise machines. No clumsy calorie-counting. No starvation. No group classes. Instead, all of this is done right in the privacy of your own home as you follow your regular daily schedule.

Now, a lifetime of youthful slimness, thanks to Slimfasting.

SPECIAL BONUS: A Special WEIGHT PROBLEM SOLVAMATIC Index enables you to locate the solution to your particular weight problem in seconds.

You are about to tap the secret of being "forever slim" with a newly rediscovered ancient technique.

Use it and help your body resist fat-building calories. From this day on, you will start to melt away unwanted pounds and inches. Slimfasting is a modern triumph over the problem of overweight.

Carlson Wade

Table of Contents

7. **The High Fiber Fast ("HFF") Way to Magic Weight Loss** 99

10 Magic Weight Losing Powers of a High Fiber Fast (100) . . . Basic High Fiber Fast Program for "Overnight" Weight Loss (101) . . . The Five-Cent Food That Is Worth a Million Dollars (103) . . . How to Use Bran in Daily Menu Planning (104) . . . How to Lose Weight on an "HFF" Meat and Potatoes Program (104) . . . How to Slimfast with Whole Grain Bread (105) . . . Easy "Seat-Slimming" High Fiber Fast Program (107) . . . Five Cents a Day Keeps the Pounds Away (108) . . . In a Nutshell (108)

8. **Slimfasting Tricks and Tips to Curb Hunger Pangs and Control Appetite** 110

Special Points (117)

9. **How to Chew Your Calories and Lose Weight with Slimfasting** . 118

How to Begin Your Slimfasting Calorie Control Program (120) . . . The "Cell-Slimming" Factor in Calorie-Chewing Slimfasting (123) . . . Official U.S. Government Recommendations for Calorie Control (124) . . . Official U.S. Government Recommendations for Calorie Control (124) . . . Table of Calories (125) . . . In Review (141)

10. **How Herbs Control Your Appetite During Slimfasting** 142

How Herbs Are All-Natural Reducing Pills (143) . . . The Herb That Erases Appetite While You Slimfast (144) . . . Herbs: How to Use Them in a Slimfasting Program (145) . . . Four Basic Types of Slimfasting Herbs (146) . . . A Garden of Slimfasting Herbs (147) . . . In Review (155)

11. **How to Use Behavior Therapy ("BT") to Stay Slim Forever and Ever** 157

Two Basic "BT" Techniques to Create Fast Weight Loss (157) . . . Seven Step Behavior Therapy Slimfasting Program for Fast "Forever Slim" Weight Loss (159) . . . How to Solve Emotional Eating Problems with Behavior Therapy (162) . . . How to Use "Thought Control" for Weight Control (163) . . . Summary (164)

12. **How a Salt-Free Slimfasting Program Creates Swift Weight Loss** 166

Salt: Cell-Fattening Cause of Overweight (166) . . . How to Plan Your Salt-Free Slimfasting Program (169) . . . How to Count Sodium Milligrams (169) . . . How a Salt-Free Program Dissolved 80 "Impossible" Pounds (178) . . . Helpful Hints for Seasoning Foods Without Salt (179) . . . How to Slimfast on Salt-Free Foods (180) . . . In Review (181)

13. **Over 40? Here are "SPC" Slimfasting Programs to Trim "Middle Age Spread"** 183

Middle Years Metabolic Slowdown (183) . . . How an "SPC" Slimfasting Program Turned "Middle Age Spread" Into an Hourglass Figure (189) . . . How "SPC" Slimfasting Adjusts Body Scales (191) . . . Summary (194)

14. **Fifteen Slimfasting Programs for Quick-Easy Weight Loss** 195

How to Follow Your Slimfasting Program (196) . . . General Guidelines for Slimfasting (200) . . . Most Important (201)

Dedication

To your new slim shape and rejuvenated body and mind

Chapter One

Slimfasting—Ancient Secret of Swift Weight Loss

Today is the first day of the rest of your slim life. Starting right now, you can begin to melt away unwanted pounds, slim down bulky extra inches from your hips and thighs, take weight off parts of your body with an ancient method that is modern science's new discovery for quick slenderness. You have heard of *fasting* as an all-natural self-cleansing method of healing used by the ancients as the ultimate cure. In our modern times, fasting can be used to help promote overall healing and also promote swift weight loss of those unsightly, unwanted, and unnecessary pounds from all parts of your body.

FASTING: KEY TO METABOLIC ADJUSTMENT

Controlled fasting, wherein certain foods are eliminated from the diet, acts as a *key* to *unlock* the sluggish metabolism that has blocked assimilation and causes weight gain. Fasting alerts and activates the process of metabolism to correct the error wherein you convert glucose to fat too rapidly and thereby gain weight. Fasting will adjust this error, help unlock the metabolic block, and thereby create more balanced endocrine secretions so that food assimilation is more efficient. *Slimfasting* adjusts your metabolic rhythm so that fats, calories, carbohydrates are "burned" more efficiently and excess pounds are "melted" instead of being stored as weight.

Fasting Is Not Starvation

Slimfasting is meant for those overweights who want to lose weight permanently *without* excessive hunger pangs, *without* being denied some favorite foods at frequent intervals, *without* the side effects usually noted with diet drugs. Most importantly, Slimfasting is NOT starvation because it uses the ancient law of "compensation" or "reparation." (Ancients called it "atonement.")

FILL UP WHILE SLIMFASTING

For example, here is a modernized method of slimfasting that helps you fill up while you slim down:

Breakfast, Day One. Have a glorious breakfast of good juicy sausages, mashed potatoes with gobs of dripping gravy, a thick wedge of apple pie with a scoop of ice cream, a cup of hot chocolate with a scoop of whipped cream topping. *Result:* The ultra-high calories and the fats and carbohydrates become stored in the form of fat and glucose to add more and more pounds of weight to your body.

Breakfast, Day Two. You now "compensate" or "atone" for the previous day's pound-adding breakfast with modified Slimfasting foods. Have a shredded lettuce and cucumber salad with a scoop of skim milk cottage cheese for dressing, a half grapefruit with a sliced peach topping, a dish of unsweetened applesauce, a cup of herb tea with lemon juice or a coffee substitute such as Postum with skim milk. *Result:* This Day Two breakfast is your "reparation" or *Slimfasting.* You have compensated for your Day One breakfast which put on pounds; your Day Two breakfast was filling but not fattening. It required a form of metabolism which helped melt away pounds.

HOW SLIMFASTING MELTS POUNDS

Your body's basic need is for calories. It needs to use calories to create fuel in the form of glucose (a simple carbohydrate). Your body's main store of glucose is in the form of glycogen in your liver. But because Day Two Breakfast had no fat and negligible calories, your metabolic system now alerts itself to your body's need for glucose.

Glucose is created by accumulated carbohydrate intake. Since Day Two Breakfast had no fat and was very low in calories and carbohydrates, your metabolic chain now starts to break down the stored up fat, calories and carbohydrates stored in your body from Day One Breakfast. During this process, there is a continued breakdown of weight-causing substances and there is comparable weight loss. In effect, on a Slimfasting program, your metabolism causes your body to literally "feed on itself" and "digest its own fat" to create swift, dramatic weight loss.

KETONES QUIET HUNGER URGE

You should not feel uncomfortable hunger on Slimfasting because the alerted metabolism steps up production of substances called *ketones.* These are substances produced from the breakdown of fats, as partial substitutes for glucose. When these ketones are released into the bloodstream, they create a soothing reaction that tends to quiet the hunger urge. So you should be able to fast while you lose weight—and feel comfortable with no annoying hunger rumbles. Slimfasting creates this metabolic process.

Fasting vs. Starvation

These are separate phenomena, completely different from each other in purpose, function and result.

1. *Fasting* is derived from the Anglo-Saxon word, *faest,* which means to "eat sparingly or to abstain from some foods."
2. *Starvation* is derived from the Old English word, *steorfan,* which means to "abstain from food entirely."

The ancients preferred to use fasting as a method of abstaining from certain types of foods and drink for longer or shorter periods of time. They never used starvation as a health method. They did not consider total food abstention as a means of improving health.

Slimfasting: Compensation without Denial of Favorite Foods. The outlined Slimfasting programs in this book show you how to use compensation so that you can remain slim while you continue enjoying most of your favorite foods.

How Elizabeth L. Uses Slimfasting for Delicious Dieting

Ever since she was a teen-ager, Elizabeth L. had waged a seemingly never-ending "battle of the bulge." She was corpulent with 40 overweight pounds that gave her unsightly jowls as well as a "spare tire" around her waistline. Many diets she tried made her feel hungry and forced her to give up her favorite foods. Elizabeth L. discovered that Slimfasting could let her "eat her cake and keep her figure at the same time." By following the simple rule of "compensation" she is able to feast upon her luscious favorite foods and lose weight. She uses Slimfasting on alternate days of the week, whenever she discovers her scales show her to be overweight.

ELIZABETH'S SLIMFASTING PROGRAM

Here is her basic program:

Sunday, Tuesday, Thursday. Eat most of your favorite foods including such indulgences as strawberry shortcake and chocolate eclairs as well as your main dish meals such as lean meat or fish.

Monday, Wednesday, Friday. Follow a simple Slimfasting program and devote each day to either fresh or cooked vegetables (or fruits), little else. Eat as many vegetables as you want in whatever combination you prefer.

Saturday. Your raw juice fasting day. Throughout the day, drink as many fruit or vegetable juices as you want, of any type that you prefer.

SECRET OF WEIGHT LOSS WITH APPETITE SATISFACTION

The favorite and high calorie foods Elizabeth L. ate during Sunday, Tuesday, Thursday are accumulating in her system as fatty tissue. These will ordinarily add pounds. But when Elizabeth L. went on a Slimfasting program during Monday, Wednesday and Friday, her metabolism broke down this food into simple molecular forms. Her metabolism used up her glucose stores and then turned to fat metabolism whereby the fatty tissues began to slim down. When Elizabeth L. followed her Saturday program of raw juice Slimfasting, all the debris and wastes were thus washed out of her system, cleansing her of accumulated toxins and melting away pound-causing fats, calories and carbohydrates.

REMAINS SLIM, SVELTE, SWEET

Elizabeth L. now remains youthfully slim, curvaceously svelte and has a sweet disposition even though she is dieting. The secret here is that the release of ketones in her bloodstream during her "off" days help keep her appetite satisfied while pounds melt away. Furthermore, during her "on" days, she can indulge in her favorite foods, a tasty delight to any dieter. Result? She appears to have won the "battle of the bulge." Her chin is firm, her waistline is almost an "hour glass" shape and her thighs are as firm as those of a teen-ager. *Added Benefit:* Regular Slimfasting has put a natural control on her appetite so that Elizabeth L. can say "no" to high-calorie foods, if she so desires. But she does indulge occasionally since she wants to "eat her cake and keep her figure at the same time." She does!

HOW TO LOOK AND FEEL NOURISHED
DURING SLIMFASTING

Nourishment during any reducing program is important. You want to look and feel adequately nourished while the pounds melt away. You do this by knowing which foods are high in essential nutrients such as protein, calcium, phosphorus, iron, and which are high (or low) in calories, fat, and carbohydrates. Select those foods for your programs which will give you a nourishing balance. Figure 1-1 tells you which foods can help you look and feel nourished during Slimfasting.

(*Note:* 100 grams = 3 1/2 ounces.)

Food, 100 g	Calo-ries	Pro-tein g	Fat g	Carbo. g	Cal-cium mg.	Phos-phorus mg.	Iron mg.
CEREAL AND FLOUR							
Corn Flakes	387	7.9	0.7	85.0	10	56	1.0
Oatmeal, Cooked	401	11.4	9.3	65.4	55	360	3.4
Wheat Flour, Sifted	344	8.5	2.0	70.9	30	220	2.2
BREAD AND CAKE							
WASA Brown Rye	370	9.0	1.5	77.0	50	350	4.0
WASA Golden Rye	370	9.0	1.5	77.0	40	250	4.0
WASA Lite Rye	370	9.0	1.5	77.0	150	400	4.0
WASA Seasoned Rye	375	9.0	3.0	76.0	40	300	4.0
Apple Pie	256	2.2	11.1	38.1	8	22	0.3
Biscuits	369	7.4	17.0	45.8	121	175	1.6
Brown Bread	211	5.5	1.3	45.6	90	160	1.9
Corn Bread	207	7.4	7.2	29.1	120	211	1.1
Cracked Wheat	263	8.7	2.2	52.1	88	128	1.1
Doughnuts, Cake	391	4.6	18.6	51.4	40	190	1.4
Fig Bars	358	3.9	5.6	75.4	78	60	1.0
French Bread	290	9.1	3.0	55.4	43	85	2.2
Gingerbread	317	3.8	10.7	52.0	68	65	2.3
Graham Crackers	384	8.0	9.4	73.3	40	149	1.5
Italian Bread	276	9.1	0.8	56.4	17	77	2.2
Muffins, Corn	314	7.1	10.1	48.1	105	169	1.7
Pancakes	231	7.1	7.0	34.1	101	139	1.3
Pizza, Cheese	236	12.0	8.3	28.3	221	195	1.0
Plain Yellow Cake	363	4.5	12.7	58.2	71	112	0.4
Pretzels	390	9.8	4.5	75.9	22	131	1.5
Raisin Bread	262	6.6	2.8	53.6	71	87	1.3

Figure 1-1

Food, 100 g	Calo-ries	Pro-tein g	Fat g	Carbo. g	Cal-cium mg.	Phos-phorus mg.	Iron mg.
Rye Bread	243	9.1	1.1	52.1	75	147	1.6
Saltines	433	9.0	12.0	71.5	21	90	1.2
Waffles	279	9.3	9.8	37.5	113	173	1.7
White Bread	269	8.7	3.2	50.4	70	87	2.4
Whole Wheat	243	10.5	3.0	47.7	99	228	2.3
DAIRY							
Cottage Cheese	106	13.6	4.2	2.9	94	152	1.3
Heavy Cream	362	2.2	37.6	3.1	75	59	Trace
Ice Cream, 12%	207	4.0	12.5	20.6	123	99	0.1
Milk	65	3.5	3.5	4.9	118	93	Trace
Skimmed Milk	36	3.6	0.1	5.1	121	95	Trace
Processed Cheese	370	23.2	30.0	1.9	697	771	0.9
Processed Cheese Spread	288	16.0	21.4	8.2	565	875	(0.6)
Yogurt, Plain	50	3.4	1.7	5.2	120	94	Trace
BUTTER AND OTHER FATS							
Butter	769	0.6	82.2	0.4	16	26	0.2
Margarine	767	0.2	82.2	0.3	4	20	0.2
Vegetable Oil	930	0	100.0	0	0	0	0
EGGS							
Whole Egg	156	12.2	11.3	0.3	60	220	2.5
Egg White	45	10.4	Trace	0.5	15	14	0.1
Egg Yolk	375	15.8	33.4	0	130	590	7.0
MEAT AND MEAT PRODUCTS							
Bacon, Cooked	611	30.4	52.0	3.2	14	224	3.3
Beef, Flank	196	30.5	7.3	0	14	150	3.8
Beef, Ground	219	27.4	11.3	0	12	230	3.5
Beef, Heart	188	31.3	5.7	0.7	6	181	5.9
Beef, Roast Chuck	327	26.0	23.9	0	11	140	3.3
Beef, Rib Roast	440	19.9	39.4	0	9	186	2.6
Beef, Round	261	28.6	15.4	0	12	250	3.5
Beef, Rump	347	23.6	27.3	0	10	197	3.1

Figure 1-1 (cont'd.)

Food, 100 g	Calo-ries	Pro-tein g	Fat g	Carbo. g	Cal-cium mg.	Phos-phorus mg.	Iron mg.
Beef, Sirloin	387	23.0	32.0	0	10	191	2.9
Chicken, Dark	176	28.0	6.3	0	13	229	1.7
Chicken, Light	166	31.6	3.4	0	11	265	1.3
Duckling	165	21.4	8.2	0	(12)	(203)	(1.3)
Game Hens	158	23.4	6.4	0	–	–	–
Ham, Boiled	234	19.0	17.0	0	11	166	2.8
Ham, Smoked	394	21.9	33.3	0	10	225	2.9
Ham, Spiced	294	15.0	24.9	1.3	9	108	2.2
Kidneys, Beef	252	33.0	12.0	0.8	18	244	13.1
Knockwurst	278	14.1	23.2	2.2	8	154	2.1
Lamb, Chop	420	19.5	37.3	0	8	150	1.1
Lamb, Leg	319	23.9	24.0	0	10	195	1.6
Lamb, Rib	492	16.9	46.5	0	7	128	0.8
Liver, Beef	229	26.4	10.6	5.3	11	476	8.8
Liver, Calves	261	29.5	13.2	4.0	13	537	14.2
Liver, Chicken	165	26.5	4.4	3.1	11	159	8.5
Liverwurst	319	14.8	27.4	2.3	10	245	5.9
Pork, Chop	387	23.5	31.8	0	10	245	3.1
Pork, Sliced	420	21.8	36.2	0	9	129	2.8
Pork, Spareribs	440	20.8	38.9	0	9	121	2.6
Salami	311	17.5	25.6	1.4	10	200	2.6
Sausage, Bologna	304	12.1	27.5	1.1	7	128	1.8
Sausage, Breakfast	476	18.1	44.2	Trace	7	162	2.4
Sausage, Frankfurter	309	12.5	27.6	1.8	7	133	1.9
Tongue, Beef	244	21.5	16.7	0.4	7	117	2.2
Turkey, Light	176	32.9	3.9	0	–	–	1.2
Turkey, Dark	203	30.0	8.3	0	–	–	2.3
Veal, Loin Chop	215	18.6	15.0	0	11	187	2.8
FISH							
Bass	196	21.5	8.5	6.7	–	–	–
Canned Tuna	197	28.8	8.2	0	(8)	234	1.9
Cod	170	28.5	5.3	0	31	274	1.0
Flounder	202	30.0	8.2	0	23	244	1.4
Haddock	165	19.6	6.4	5.8	40	247	1.2
Halibut	171	25.2	7.0	0	16	248	0.8

Figure 1-1 (cont'd.)

Food, 100 g	Calo-ries	Pro-tein g	Fat g	Carbo. g	Cal-cium mg.	Phos-phorus mg.	Iron mg.
Mackerel	236	21.8	15.8	0	6	280	1.2
Ocean Perch	227	19.0	13.3	6.8	33	226	1.3
Pompano	166	18.8	9.5	0	—	—	—
Porgy	112	19.0	3.4	0	54	250	—
Red Snapper	93	19.8	0.9	0	16	214	0.8
Salmon	182	27.0	7.4	0	—	414	1.2
Smelt	200	18.4	13.5	0	358	370	1.7
Sole	79	16.7	0.8	0	12	195	0.8
Swordfish	174	28.0	6.0	0	27	275	1.3
Whitefish, Smoked	155	20.9	7.3	0	22	274	—
SHELLFISH							
Clam, Raw	80	11.1	0.9	5.9	69	151	7.5
Crabmeat	93	17.3	1.9	0.5	43	175	0.8
Lobster	95	18.7	1.5	0.3	65	192	0.8
Oysters, Raw	66	8.4	1.8	3.4	94	143	5.5
Shrimp	116	24.2	1.1	0.7	115	263	3.1
FRUITS							
Apples	58	0.2	0.6	14.5	7	10	0.3
Apricots	51	1.0	0.2	12.8	17	23	0.5
Avocados	167	2.1	16.4	6.3	10	42	0.6
Bananas	85	1.1	0.2	22.2	8	26	0.7
Blueberries	62	0.7	0.5	15.3	15	13	1.0
Cherries, Sweet	70	1.3	0.3	17.4	22	19	0.4
Dates, Dried	274	2.2	0.5	72.9	59	63	3.0
Figs, Dried	274	4.3	1.3	69.1	126	77	3.0
Grapefruit	41	0.5	0.1	10.6	16	16	0.4
Grapes	69	1.3	1.0	15.7	16	12	0.4
Lemon Juice	25	0.5	0.2	8.0	7	10	0.2
Oranges	40	1.0	0.2	12.2	41	20	0.4
Peaches	38	0.6	0.1	9.7	9	19	0.5
Pears	61	0.7	0.4	15.3	8	11	0.3
Pineapples	52	0.4	0.2	13.7	17	8	0.5
Plums	48	0.5	0.2	12.3	12	18	0.5
Prunes, Cooked	119	1.0	0.3	31.4	24	37	1.8
Raisins	289	2.5	0.2	77.4	62	101	3.5
Raspberries	57	1.2	0.5	13.6	22	22	0.9
Strawberries	37	0.7	0.5	8.4	21	21	1.0

Figure 1-1 (cont'd.)

Food, 100 g	Calo-ries	Pro-tein g	Fat g	Carbo. g	Cal-cium mg.	Phos-phorus mg.	Iron mg.
Watermelon	26	0.5	0.2	6.4	7	10	0.5
VEGETABLES							
Asparagus	20	2.2	0.2	3.6	21	50	0.6
Beans, Lima	111	7.6	0.5	19.8	47	121	2.5
Beans, Green	25	1.6	0.2	5.4	50	37	0.6
Broccoli	26	3.1	0.3	4.5	88	62	0.8
Brussel Sprouts	36	4.2	0.4	6.4	32	72	1.1
Cabbage	18	1.0	0.2	4.0	42	17	0.3
Cauliflower	22	2.3	0.2	4.1	21	42	0.7
Celery, Raw	17	0.9	0.1	3.9	39	28	0.3
Corn	83	3.2	1.0	18.8	3	89	0.6
Lettuce, Iceberg	13	0.9	0.1	2.9	20	22	0.5
Mushrooms, Raw	28	2.7	0.3	4.4	6	116	0.8
Onions, Cooked	29	1.2	0.1	6.5	24	29	0.4
Peas	71	5.4	0.4	12.1	23	99	1.8
Peppers, Green, Raw	22	1.2	0.2	4.8	9	22	0.7
Potato, Sweet, Baked	141	2.1	0.5	32.5	40	58	0.9
Potato, White, Boiled	65	1.9	0.1	14.5	6	42	0.5
Spinach	23	3.0	0.3	3.6	83	38	2.2
Squash, Summer	14	0.9	0.1	3.1	25	25	0.4
Tomatoes, Raw	22	1.1	0.2	4.7	13	27	0.5
Turnips	23	0.8	0.2	4.9	35	24	0.4
Watercress	19	2.2	0.3	3.0	151	54	1.7
Yams, Raw	101	2.1	0.2	23.2	20	69	0.6
Zucchini	12	1.0	0.1	2.5	25	25	0.4
MISCELLA-NEOUS							
Chocolate Milk	85	3.4	3.4	11.0	111	94	0.2
Coffee	1	Trace	Trace	Trace	2	4	0.1
Gelatin + Fruit	67	1.3	0.1	16.4	–	–	–
Honey	304	0.3	0	82.3	5	6	0.5
Milk Chocolate	528	4.4	35.1	57.9	94	142	1.4
Pudding, Vanilla	111	3.5	3.9	15.9	117	91	Trace
Sugar	385	0	0	99.5	85	0	0.1
Tea	2	–	Trace	0.4	Trace	–	Trace

Figure 1-1 (cont'd.)

FASTING—ANCIENT ALL-PURPOSE HEALER

Fasting was used by the ancients as an all-purpose healer. Religious fasting is of early origin, antedating recorded history. Partial or total abstinence from certain kinds of foods, at stated seasons, prevailed in ancient Assyria, Persia, Babylon, Scythia, Greece, Rome, India, Nineveh, Palestine, China, in northern Europe among the Druids and in America among the Indians.

MYSTICAL POWER OF FASTING

At the very dawn of civilization the Ancient Mysteries, a secret worship or wisdom religion that flourished for thousands of years in Egypt, India, Greece, Persia, Thrace, Scandinavia and the Gothic and Celtic nations, prescribed and practiced fasting as part of mystical rites. They reportedly believed that they derived strange powers of strength from periodic fasting.

The Druid religion among the Celtic peoples required a long probationary period of fasting and prayer before the candidate could advance. A fast of fifty days was required in the Mithraic religion in Persia. Fasting was common to all the "mystery religions," which were all quite similar to the Egyptian mystery religions and were probably derived from these. Moses, who was learned in "all the wisdom of Egypt" is said to have fasted for more than 120 days on Mount Sinai.

Note: The ancients did not abstain from all foods for those long periods of time. Rather, they would subsist entirely upon raw fruits or raw vegetables during their fasting. This gave them nourishment during their fasting.

FASTING AS A CURE

The mystery religion of Tyre, which was represented in Judea some 2000 years ago in a secret society known as the Essenes, also prescribed fasting as a cure. They would prescribe "fruit fasts" or "vegetable fasts" or "grain fasts" or "milk fasts" as means of healing as well as slimming down the corpulent.

In the first century A.D., there lived in Alexandria, Egypt, an ascetic sect called Therapeutae, who resembled the Essenes. They borrowed much from the Cabala, a secret esoteric doctrine which prescribed fasting as a means of improving health and curing almost all known ailments. The Therapeutae used the principles outlined in the Cabala, as well as the Pythagorian and Orphic systems and prescribed fasting as a curative measure for weight problems and related disorders.

BIBLE RECOMMENDATIONS FOR FASTING

To restore health, which begins with a youthfully slim shape, the ancients recommended periodic fasting. The Bible tells of many such fasts. Moses fasted for 40 days. (Exodus 24:18, 34:28.) Elijah fasted for 40 days. (1 Kings 19:8.) David fasted for 7 days. (2 Samuel 12:16.) Jesus fasted for 40 days. (Matthew 4:2.) Fasting twice a week is recommended in the gospels. (Luke 18:12, Matthew 17:21.) All of Judea fasted regularly. (2 Chronicles 20:3.)

The Bible cautions against fasting for mere notoriety. (Matthew 6:17, 18.) The Bible advises those who fast not to wear a sad countenance. (Matthew 6:16.) The Bible suggests that you find pleasure in fasting and to perform your work. (Isaiah 58:3.) The Bible suggests that certain fasts be fasts of gladness. (Zachariah 8:19.)

FASTING BECOMES PART OF HISTORY

Fasting has always been a regular practice among the nations of the Far East, especially amongst the East Indians. Among the early Christians, fasting was one of the rites of purification and self-healing. The early Church had rules of fasting which are similar to those of Slimfasting as described in this book. Namely, during certain times, the eating of meat was forbidden; however, eggs and dairy products could be used. In earlier times, fasting was described as having only one full meal in one particular day.

The early practice of fasting until sundown is similar to that of the Moslems during their fast of the month of Ramadan. It is said that the Archangel Michael appeared to a certain priest of Sipponte, after the latter had spent a year in fasting. We should understand that this "year of fasting" certainly did not mean that all food was eliminated. Instead, certain heavier foods of meat origin were omitted while fruits, vegetables and grains were enjoyed for better health.

Fasting also formed parts of the religious observances of the Aztecs and Toltecs of Mexico, the Incas of Peru, and of other American tribes. Fasting was also practiced by the Pacific Islanders. There are records of fasting in China and Japan, even before their contact with Buddhism.

Almost all civilizations in all parts of the world have recommended the use of periodic fasting as a means of helping the body cleanse itself and become more youthful with a slimmer figure.

FASTING PRESCRIBED BY DOCTORS

As an all-natural weight-losing program, fasting has been used by physicians for many decades. It was prescribed for those patients who wanted to have an all-natural means for melting away pounds and inches. It was especially desirable for patients who found it both difficult and time-consuming to lose weight on other programs. Reports about the success of fasting have appeared in many of the world's leading medical and scientific journals. This led to fasting being regarded as an effective way to help weight come off and be kept off in a reasonably short time length. The public as well as the medical world has become aware of fasting as an easy and speedy way to shed pounds and inches. So it is that overweights are now aware of fasting as much as they are aware of calories in their quest for slimming down.

FASTING USED IN HEALTH SPAS

Whether in the places known as "fat farms" or "beauty farms" or exclusive "health spas," overweights have used fasting for more than half a century. Folks who emerged slim and youthful from this type of resort have helped spread the knowledge about fasting so that it is almost a household word. Many overweights use fasting right in their own homes, following the same programs as used in exclusive and costly health spas. These are the programs outlined in this book.

HOW TO TAKE OFF "INCH AFTER INCH"
WITH SLIMFASTING + BEHAVIOR THERAPY

A combination of Slimfasting with behavior therapy self-treatment can readjust your physiological-emotional appetite control centers so that you can actually satisfy yourself with smaller portions of food as you take off unsightly inches.

Secretary Uses Combo Plan for Quick Slimming

Marge A. was a secretary with a weight problem. She had tried the "round robin" of different reducing programs. She would lose pounds, true, but she would gain them right back because she made up for lost meals with overeating. She had tried motivation or so-called "behavior therapy" but she could not "think thin" long enough to lose those four unwanted inches around her waistline and hips. Furthermore, Marge A. complained that other diets often left her hungry, not to mention tired. What to do?

The combination plan she selected called for using a Slimfasting program *together* with behavior therapy. When she used this simple combo plan, she began to lose unwanted and bulging "inches" while feeling fully satisfied insofar as her eating urges were concerned.

Here is Marge A.'s combo plan:

SLIMFASTING PROGRAM

She decided upon a 1200 calorie-per-day program. She selected an assortment of foods from Figure 1-1, emphasizing those foods that were high in protein, calcium, phosphorus and iron. These four nutrients satisfied her appetite so that she no longer felt hunger pangs or "knots" that demanded food.

Marge A. could eat *any* of the foods (including ice cream, apple pie, vanilla pudding) provided they did not tip the balance of being over 1200 calories per day. To provide good nutrition, Marge A. ate these hitherto "no-no" foods in small quantities but emphasized more nutritious foods in the list. The secretary found that on this combo program, she would lose inch after inch from her waistline and hips. Yet Marge A. needed self-help behavior therapy to enable her to remain on this delicious Slimfasting program.

DO-IT-YOURSELF BEHAVIOR THERAPY PROGRAM

Marge A. used self-help behavior therapy so she would be satisfied with occasional *smaller* portions of apple pie a la mode with chocolate syrup. To "re-educate" her appestat (appetite control center in the brain), she would *self-motivate* herself with these methods of behavior-therapy:

1. Put a smaller portion of a high-calorie food on a small plate. A small wedge of pie on a smaller plate makes it look very large. This offers as much eating satisfaction and joy as if it were, in reality, a larger portion.

2. Before eating, wait a few moments. Make a ritual out of eating. Wrap all utensils in a napkin. Wait about two or three minutes before beginning. Slowly unwrap utensils. Whenever you put food in your mouth, put down the utensil. Let it remain there until you have slowly chewed and swallowed the food. Then pick up the utensil and repeat the slow process until you have finished the meal. This, too, makes smaller portions appear to be as satisfying as larger portions.

3. If you feel the urge to eat between meals, find something else to do: Read a book. Try needlework. Play games with somebody or even by yourself. Take a shower or bubble bath. If possible, get out of the house for a walk. Go to a movie. Divert your mind, and the feeling of hunger should pass.

"INCH AFTER INCH" SHRINKS AWAY

This combination plan of Slimfasting + behavior therapy worked for Marge A. The secretary used a tape measure around her waist and hips almost daily. Joyfully, she noted that the unwanted inches began to shrink away. After only 24 days on this combo plan, Marge A. lost four inches around her midriff and hips. No rigorous dieting. No hunger pains. No denial of most of her favorite foods. No tired feeling. No weakness. No "tired" blood. The inches shrank away and she had a lovely figure.

Marge A. could remain *slim forever* on this combination plan. She could also enjoy a wide variety of different foods from the chart and have a "feast" while "fasting" her way to a youthful figure.

ANCIENT SECRET = SCIENTIFIC FACT

The ancients prescribed fasting as a slimming-healing treatment. They lacked our modern scientific terminology, but they knew that it worked. For many ancient sects, it was a secret way to self-rejuvenation.

In modern times, we know that Slimfasting is a scientific fact. Here is how it works:

Nutrition or metabolism does not cease during a fast because nutrition is life. The purpose of Slimfasting is not to suspend metabolism but to *alert-activate-amplify* its power. This "triple A" power is the key to slimming down.

Even when food is limited or restricted, your body's organs and systems must continue to eat. Therefore, they turn to the only source of internal nutriment: your *adipose tissues.*

It is a scientific fact that much stubborn fat is "locked" in your adipose or fatty tissues. You have millions of these cells and tissues that are overburdened with accumulated fat. During Slimfasting, your metabolism turns to these "fat cells" or *adipose tissues* and takes out accumulated fats, calories and carbohydrates, transporting them to your body's organs and systems for nourishment. This helps to reduce your "fat cells" and correspondingly help reduce your body.

Slimfasting uses this ancient secret for natural reducing. Your "fat cells" cannot be slimmed down through metabolism if you continue to eat heavily. The more you eat, the more your adipose tissues "gain weight." Furthermore, your metabolism takes fats, calories and carbohydrates from daily food *without* tapping the reserves in your fat cells. When your metabolism bypasses your fat cells, they increase in size—and so do you!

To enable your metabolism to get at the "locked in" fats, calories and carbohydrates in your adipose tissues, you have to reduce your intake of food. When you do this, your metabolism is forced to seek nourishment from the body's reserves and your fat cells are the primary targets. Withdrawing weight from the cells, the secret of the ancient technique of healthy reducing, is known in modern science as Slimfasting.

HIGHLIGHTS

1. Lose unwanted pounds and inches with an ancient method known as fasting. It is the key to metabolic adjustment and overall slimming.

2. Fill up while Slimfasting on the "compensation" or "atonement" method by enjoying luscious foods one day and then low-calorie good foods the next day. Strike this balance and you can reduce while eating under a Slimfasting program.

3. Slimfasting is not starvation. It does not deny your favorite foods. You can "have your cake and eat it too," as did Elizabeth L. on a simple Slimfasting program that firmed up her chin and gave her an hour-glass figure like a teenager.

4. Look and feel well-nourished without hunger pains or nutritional deficiency by selecting a variety of calorie-carbohydrate-fat *regulated* foods from the listed charts. Emphasize those high in other nutrients.

5. Fasting was prescribed as an all-purpose healer for thousands of years by the ancients.

6. Slimfasting + behavior therapy helped secretary Marge A. take off "inch after inch" on a special 1200 calorie per day program. She enjoyed ice cream, apple pie, vanilla pudding—and good health—while she lost four inches from her waist and hips!

7. The ancients considered fasting as a secret cure. Modern science recognizes it as a proven fact. Slimfasting works by enabling your metabolism to "eat" stored up weight from your "fat cells" or adipose tissues and melt away pounds and reduce inches.

Chapter Two

How to Reshape,
Revitalize, Rejuvenate
Your Body with Slimfasting

The ancients looked upon fasting as more than a natural way to lose weight. They regarded fasting as a method of self-rejuvenation. After following several days or periodic occasions of controlled fasting, they emerged looking and feeling more youthful. In modern times, we recognize that fasting can help stimulate sluggish metabolic-circulatory processes and create a form of self-cleansing of the billions of body cells that promote the look and feel of youth.

SLIMFASTING—WHAT IT DOES FOR YOU

With reduced food intake, the body begins to metabolize its own reserves. Basically, your fatty tissue is a storage site for toxic wastes that are not ordinarily (or easily) eliminated if you eat full meals daily. The more extra fat you carry, the more toxins you carry. Slimfasting will help lose extra fat together with the unwanted toxins.

SLIMFASTING PROMOTES INTERNAL CLEANSING

During a Slimfasting program, your body is able to become "cleansed" since the task of digesting food is eased or temporarily halted. During the process of digestion, your body is busy breaking food down into simple molecular forms to provide energy. Your body transforms proteins into amino acids, carbohydrates into sugars, fats into fatty acids. This occupies much of the efforts of your digestive process. But during Slimfasting, a self-rejuvenation process takes place. Slimfasting enables fat metabolism to occur outside your digestive tract; this eases the burden on your digestive organs. Now your body is able to begin the process of *autolysis* or "self-loosening" of the accumulated wastes and help cast them out of your system through your eliminative channels. Within one or two days, much of the stored up toxic wastes in your fatty tissues have been subjected to autolysis and are being washed out of your system, along with excess weight. This promotes a feeling of internal and external revitalization and an appearance of rejuvenation.

SLIMFASTING IS A NATURAL ENERGY DIET

Millions of overweight folks have tried different types of reducing diets with varying degrees of success. For them, a special low-calorie or low-carbohydrate program can melt away unwanted pounds and slim down bulging inches. But there are many who complain that many reducing diets leave them feeling weak, listless, without energy. For those who want to feel energetic and "alive" during dieting, Slimfasting is a welcome program. It does not call for the total abstinence from food for extended periods of time. It calls for reduction and "compensation" plan. That is, when you use Slimfasting, you eat less and less of your favorite foods. Then, if you indulge in your favorite chocolate cake, you "compensate" by either skipping a meal or enjoying a meal consisting only of crisp, raw vegetables. This helps "compensate" for the added calories stored up with the cake.

SLIMFASTING VS. STARVATION

It is important to emphasize again that Slimfasting is not starvation which is an energy-draining and unhealthy alternative. During Slimfasting, you eat moderately or drink moderately and your body continues to store valuable nutrients. During this Slimfasting program, your body turns to feed upon its own reserves; it will draw upon fat, muscle, blood, water, tissues.

VITAL ORGANS PROTECTED

During Slimfasting, with modest intake of food and beverages, your vital body organs such as your brain, spinal cord, bones, etc., are sustained and protected. It is only when the body is denied food for a very long period of time that the process of starvation begins. A supervised Slimfasting program calls for reduction or eliminaton of foods for a brief amount of time or until the body reserves have been used up. At this time, there is a feeling of healthy hunger, a clear tongue, bright, shining eyes, youthful skin, alert muscles, more limbered up arms and legs. Slimfasting promotes this internal cleanliness without depriving you of important mental and physical energy since it protects your vital organs.

SLIMFASTING IS A NATURAL REJUVENATION PROGRAM

Your body has its own built-in protective system whereby surplus protein, fats, carbohydrates and calories are consumed during the process of autolysis, then cast out through the eliminative channels, creating sparkling cleanliness internally and externally.

PROTEIN-SPARING MECHANISM

During Slimfasting, your body brings a special protein-sparing mechanism into play. Ordinarily, your body requires from 100 to 150 grams of glucose each day. During Slimfasting, with a reduction or elimination of food, this amount may not be available. Therefore, your metabolism now draws some glucose from your liver's reserve of glycogen. When this has been used up, your metabolism now turns to the protein stored in your muscles.

Your metabolism takes this stored up protein and uses it to rebuild and replenish the billions of damaged tissues and cells throughout your body. Your metabolism uses this protein to revitalize and "wash" your bloodstream and also to repair your internal organs. Your body has a "stop button" mechanism whereby sufficient protein still remains in your skeletal muscles so that they do not "starve." But if total abstinence from food occurs for more than ten days, without medical supervision, then the "stop button" loses its power. A short-circut occurs and precious reserves of protein are withdrawn from the skeletal muscles and starvation occurs.

CONTROLLED SLIMFASTING IS HEALTHFUL

Slimfasting programs should be controlled, planned for, followed carefully and for brief amounts of time. During Slimfasting, your body takes steps to conserve its supplies of protein. Special hormones alert a special "rejuvenation switch" in your system and your brain promptly adapts ketones (substances released in the bloodstream during Slimfasting) as a substitute source of energy. This explains why many folks have found Slimfasting effective as a reducing program: It leaves them feeling energetic, strong, alert, even while dieting!

HOW TO BEGIN YOUR SLIMFASTING PROGRAM

Here's a special set of instructions to guide you into your Slimfasting program.

Setting Your Weight Goals

Are you overweight? Look in a mirror! That's the quickest way to see if you're overweight. If you want to be more precise, check your present weight against the height/weight/sex scales in Figure 2-1.

CALCULATING YOUR PROPER WEIGHT

There are two rule-of-thumb systems for calculating your ideal weight. (1) Assume an average weight of 100 to 110 pounds. Add 5 pounds for each inch you measure over five feet. (2) Specialists believe that your weight at 30 years is the ideal weight to maintain for the remainder of your life if your weight at age 30 is ideal.

Eight Starter Steps for Slimfasting

A trim figure is the dream of almost everyone. But it need not remain a dream. With Slimfasting, it's within the grasp of everyone. Slimfasting requires the application of a few simple principles. Success depends upon how serious you are. Here are eight starter steps for Slimfasting:

1. *Check* your ideal weight from the table in this chapter.
2. *Determine* that you *will* reduce to that weight.
3. *Begin today* on a definite regimen of weight reduction. Remember, tomorrow may be too late.
4. *Use common sense.* Don't try to achieve the ideal weight in a few hours or a day. It will take a liitle patience, perseverance, effort to undo the harm that has been occurring for perhaps half your lifetime.
5. *Keep* a set of bathroom scales. Weigh in daily; preferably without clothes, and at the same time each day.
6. *Don't be discouraged* if progress is slow at first. Doggedly stick to the Slimfasting program.
7. *Work out* a sensible Slimfasting diet plan from those presented in this book.
8. *Remember* you *will* succeed with effort. Millions have!

STEP-BY-STEP GUIDE TO SLIMFASTING

Here's a step-by-step guide to help you ease into Slimfasting and enjoy this quick "pounds off" way to youthful slimness:

"IDEAL WEIGHT"

Tables for Height and Weight Without Clothing*

		WOMEN						MEN			
FT.	IN.	15 YRS	20 YRS	25 YRS	30 YRS	FT.	IN.	15 YRS	20 YRS	25 YRS	30 YRS
4	8	90 *100* 113	95 *105* 117	97 *108* 122	100 *111* 125	4	11	92 *102* 114	101 *112* 126	105 *117* 131	109 *121* 136
4	9	91 *101* 114	96 *107* 119	99 *110* 124	102 *113* 127	5	0	94 *104* 117	103 *114* 128	107 *119* 134	111 *123* 138
4	10	92 *102* 115	98 *109* 123	101 *112* 126	104 *115* 129	5	1	96 *107* 120	105 *117* 131	109 *121* 136	113 *125* 140
4	11	94 *104* 117	100 *111* 125	103 *114* 128	105 *117* 132	5	2	99 *110* 124	108 *120* 135	112 *124* 139	115 *128* 144
5	0	96 *107* 120	103 *114* 128	104 *116* 131	107 *119* 134	5	3	102 *113* 127	111 *123* 138	115 *128* 144	118 *131* 147
5	1	99 *110* 122	105 *117* 132	107 *119* 134	110 *122* 137	5	4	105 *117* 131	114 *127* 143	119 *132* 148	122 *135* 152
5	2	102 *113* 127	108 *120* 135	111 *123* 138	113 *125* 141	5	5	109 *121* 136	118 *131* 147	123 *136* 153	125 *139* 156
5	3	104 *116* 131	111 *123* 138	113 *126* 142	116 *129* 145	5	6	113 *125* 140	122 *135* 152	126 *140* 157	129 *143* 161
5	4	108 *120* 135	113 *126* 142	116 *129* 145	119 *132* 149	5	7	116 *129* 145	125 *139* 156	130 *144* 162	132 *147* 165
5	5	112 *124* 140	117 *130* 146	120 *133* 149	123 *136* 153	5	8	120 *133* 149	129 *143* 161	133 *148* 166	136 *151* 170
5	6	115 *128* 144	121 *134* 151	123 *137* 154	126 *140* 158	5	9	123 *137* 154	132 *147* 165	137 *152* 171	141 *156* 175
5	7	119 *132* 149	124 *138* 155	127 *141* 158	130 *144* 162	5	10	128 *142* 159	136 *151* 170	141 *157* 176	145 *161* 181
5	8	122 *136* 153	127 *141* 159	131 *145* 163	133 *148* 167	5	11	132 *147* 165	141 *156* 175	146 *162* 182	150 *167* 188
5	9	126 *140* 158	131 *145* 163	134 *149* 167	136 *151* 170	6	0	137 *152* 171	145 *161* 181	151 *168* 189	156 *173* 194
5	10	131 *145* 163	134 *149* 168	137 *152* 171	140 *155* 174	6	1	141 *157* 176	150 *166* 186	157 *174* 195	161 *179* 201
5	11	135 *150* 168	139 *154* 173	140 *156* 176	143 *159* 179	6	2	146 *162* 182	154 *171* 192	161 *179* 201	167 *185* 208

*Table from Life Extension Institute of New York City.

THREE WEIGHTS GIVEN

1. Middle figures *in italics* for medium build (medium bone weight for height); average weight.
2. Upper figures for slender build (light bone weight for height; 10 per cent reduction from average weight.
3. Lower figures for large frame (heavy bone weight for height)? 12 1/2 per cent added to average weight. (The ideal weight for 30 years should be maintained throughout life.)

Figure 2-1

Day Before Your Fast. Prepare yourself for Slimfasting by cutting down on portions of your usual foods the day *before* you begin. If you are a "sugarholic" and must have your sweet pastry with your coffee, go ahead and indulge—but eat a half portion. This will prepare your metabolism for your Slimfasting experience.

First Day of Your Fast. Devote the entire day to the eating of fresh raw vegetables prepared as a salad, for munching, and as a main meal. Take no other foods. Drink at least two or three quarts of water during your first day and continue drinking as much water as possible throughout your Slimfasting program. *Benefit:* The raw vegetables are prime sources of vitamins, minerals, essential enzymes which are taken up by your metabolism to help digest and loosen accumulated fats so they can be washed out of your body. Water is most essential on any Slimfasting program. Water will flush out the toxins and waste materials that accumulate when fatty tissue is being "burned." Water protects your body organs against dehydration. Water will relieve any "hunger pangs" that may be felt at the very start of your Slimfasting.

Second Day of Your Fast. Devote the entire day to the eating of fresh raw fruits prepared as a salad, for munching, as a main meal. You may use some slightly steamed fruits for a different taste and a feeling of soothing warmth for your digestive system. Continue drinking as much water as is comfortably possible. *Benefit:* The raw fruits are high in Vitamin C and many minerals which are needed to repair the billions of body cells and tissues as well as your internal organs. The water is also needed to help flush out accumulated debris from your body. Since your fat intake is reduced on this program, your metabolism begins to break up the stored amount of fat in your adipose tissues and the slimming process is well underway. The water will wash out this fatty debris.

Third Day of Your Fast. Now you may change to a menu of steamed or baked vegetables in the form of a salad or a main dish. If you boil vegetables, use as little water as possible to preserve nutrients; keep the kettle covered and boil only long enough for the vegetables to become tender. Continue drinking all the water you can comfortably enjoy. *Benefit:* The steamed or cooked vegetables offer you roughage or cellulose which will help maintain intestinal mobility so that accumulated blocks of waste and debris can be further removed. The water will liquefy any "stubborn deposits" that need to be eliminated. This further reduces weight while cleansing your internal organs and giving you a feeling of youthful alertness.

Fourth Day of Your Fast. Enjoy a combination of fresh, raw vegetables and cooked vegetables. You may also finish your vegetable meal with fruit dessert. Again, continue drinking adequate amounts of water. *Benefit:* The vegetables and the fruit are prime sources of vitamins, minerals, enzymes, roughage which will nourish your system *without* adding any fats. The water will act as a transport or carrier of discharge, removing the fats and the wastes, thereby slimming down your body while creating what the ancients regarded as *youthful purification.*

Fifth (Final) Day of Your Fast. Enjoy both fresh and cooked vegetables, fresh and cooked fruits and add a variety of desired vegetable and fruit juices. Drink freely. You may also drink water, in addition to the plant juices. *Benefit:* A double-barreled reaction occurs with the nutrients in the vegetables and fruits. They are activated by the enzymes and nutrients in the raw juices and work to "dissolve" and "scrape" away accumulated sludge and debris to complete the reducing and cleansing effect.

How to Ease Out of Your Slimfasting Program

Do not shock your system by suddenly going from a "fast" to a "feast." This will upset your metabolism. This will also contradict all the benefits of Slimfasting and your weight will zoom up again. Instead, follow this guideline:

First Day after Your Fast. Slowly start adding yogurt, non-processed and natural dairy products such as cottage cheese, farmer cheese. Continue enjoying fruits and vegetables and their juices as well as water.

Second Day after Your Fast. Now add broiled fish, whole grains in skim milk and very thin slices of whole grain bread. Continue with fruits and vegetables and their juices and as much water as you comfortably enjoy.

Third Day after Your Fast. Now add baked or broiled chicken or turkey, with large amounts of fruits, vegetables and juices.

Fourth Day after Your Fast. Add lean broiled meat and continue taking large amounts of fruits, vegetables and juices.

By now you have eased out of your Slimfasting. Your skin should be brighter, your eyes should sparkle, your arms and legs should move with more youthful agility, you should feel lighter in more ways than one. Check your scale. Tape measure your waistline. Then check it against your desired weight. If you need to lose more weight or take off more inches, then plan to go on a Slimfasting program at least one week a month. Finally, DO NOT go on an "eating binge" after your Slimfasting. Instead, adjust yourself to satisfying amounts of foods that nourish but do not overburden your system. This is your key to a slim and youthful body and mind.

How Slimfasting Trimmed a Waistline
from 54 to 35 in Three Weeks

Michael B. did not become overweight in a short while. His expanding waistline was stuffed into a 54 inch belt, and it threatened to increase in girth! But Michael B. was impatient and wanted to lose his weight in a short span of time. He had frequent dizzy spells. His blood pressure was very high. His love for sweets threatened to give him diabetes, a condition frequently accompanying overweight. Michael B. knew he had to lose weight—and he wanted to lose it fast!

OTHER DIETS HAD "YO-YO" EFFECT

Michael B. had lost many pounds and even two dozen inches from his waistline on other diets. True, they did work for him, as they did for others. But Michael B. was a compulsive eater, forever beset with hunger pangs, real or imagined. So he succumbed to the "yo-yo" effect. He lost enormous weight on those diets, but his peculiar "hunger urge" made him ravenous, so that after completing the diet he went on "eating orgies" and not only gained back lost pounds—but gained new and more unwanted pounds!

"TRY SLIMFASTING BECAUSE IT WORKS"

So said Michael B.'s physician. He told him to go on a Slimfasting diet because many doctors recommend such a program to their overweights. So do many weight-loss specialists who have reported that even the most stubborn weight can be shed on a fasting program. They have reported seeing results from various health spas and from published medical documents. These same Slimfasting programs can be followed at home with similar weight-losing results. So when Michael B.'s doctor suggested that he follow this same program, he decided it was the answer to his stubborn overweight problem.

THE SUCCESS OF THE HIGH-PROTEIN, LOW CARBO-CAL SLIMFASTING PLAN

Since Michael B. could not conquer his compulsive eating urge, he turned to a simple, tasty plan which allowed him to eat high-protein foods but eliminated or reduced carbohydrate and high calorie foods.

Chews His Way to Reduced Waistline. The Slimfasting plan let Michael B. eat lean meats, especially turkey and chicken. He reduced his intake of fruits and vegetables. In his particular case, he needed to drastically cut down carbohydrates from all sources. (Later he would resume eating plant foods when his metabolism was balanced and could assimilate carbohydrates.) He eliminated grains. Michael B. boasted that on his Slimfasting plan, he could indulge in all the meats he wanted but he had to chew them very thoroughly before swallowing. He was also told to drink as much water as he could comfortably enjoy. He could also drink herb tea (without sugar) or a coffee substitute such as Postum (with skim milk, but no sugar).

Loses 7 Inches in 7 Days. During the first days of this easy and delicious Slimfasting plan, Michael B. saw his waistline go down. He lost 7 inches within 7 days.

Reaches a Slim 35 Inch Wastline in 21 Days. By the time Michael reached the 21st day of his Slimfasting plan, his waistline was an amazingly youthful 35 inches. Furthermore, he felt his compulsive eating urge and been "licked" and now he could enjoy many of his favorite foods but in normal quantities. His 35 inch waistline would remain a slim 35 inches!

Basic Health Improves. He no longer had dizzy spells. His blood pressure was satisfactory. The threat of diabetes was over. Now he could enjoy an occasional strawberry shortcake (his favorite dessert) and a martini. He had successfully conquered his compulsive eating urge.

WHY THIS SLIMFASTING PROGRAM REMOVED STUBBORN POUNDS

Michael B. had an expanding waistline and extra pounds because of his uncontrollable eating urge. Other diets could not correct the *cause* of his runaway appetite. But Slimfasting worked because when he cut down or eliminated his intake of carbohydrates and calories, his metabolism could secrete compounds known as *ketones.*

Basically, ketones are byproducts of metabolized fatty acids. When these ketones pour into the bloodstream, they act as natural appetite suppressants. *Ketones are released strongly into the bloodstream only when you are on a low- or no-carbohydrate and calorie Slimfasting program.* You may continue eating your favorite protein foods (meat, fish, eggs, dairy products, poultry) to your satisfaction.

For Michael B., once the ketones went into his bloodstream, his appetite started to shrink; he felt less of an eating urge. He ate his favorite meats but in sharply reduced amounts and with great satisfaction! During the Slimfasting program, the ketones acted as an *appetite-block* and this helped him lose stubborn pounds and shrink inches from his waistline.

A high-protein but low- or no-carbohydrate and calorie Slim-fasting program can help the scales (and waistline) go down, thanks to the ketone response.

"Slim Down or Ship Out"

Edgar R. looked much older than his 40 years because of his weight. His skin developed wrinkled furrows. Bags appeared beneath his bleary eyes. He moved with the stiff and jerky motions of an elderly person. His actions were slow. There were times when he had to hold on to the arms of his chair in order to stand up!

"LOSE WEIGHT OR YOU'RE FIRED!"

His superiors were displeased that Edgar R. was so overweight. Company medical reports indicated his 45 extra pounds posed a serious health risk. Edgar R. was told to lose weight or he might be fired. The company president was more blunt—he told Edgar to "slim down or ship out!"

A SWEET SLIMFASTING PLAN THAT ERASED OVER 50 POUNDS

Edgar R. had previously lost many pounds on other highly recognized and reputable reducing diets. But Edgar R. loved to eat candies (chocolate covered raisin bars were his favorite) and take a bottle of beer with his meals. Other diets would have worked it he could have refrained from the candy-and-beer habit. He selected a very simple Slimfasting plan that would permit him to indulge in his habit but lose weight at the same time. Here is the amazingly simple yet even more amazingly successful Slimfasting plan that took over 50 pounds from his body.

The "Even Day Slimfasting Plan": Edgar R. was told that on the even days of the month (that is, the 2nd, 4th, 6th, 8th, etc., right down to the 30th day of the month) he would follow this Slimfasting plan—to devote the entire day to the eating of only fresh raw vegetables, in any form and in any quantity. He was told not to eat anything else during the even days of the month. He could drink all the water he wanted.

The "Odd Day Slimfasting Plan": On every odd day of the month (the 1st, 3rd, 5th, 7th, right down to the 31st day) he could have most of his favorite foods, even his favorite sweet and his beer.

LOSES 50+ POUNDS, RESTORES YOUTHFUL HEALTH

By the time he finished on the 31st day, he had lost fifty-*plus* pounds, his waistline melted to a healthier 36. His bulbous chin and heavy cheeks flattened out. He walked with a youthful bounce. He displayed amazing energy for a young 40 year old executive. His eyes were bright. His reflexes were alert. The Even-Odd Day Slimfasting Plan had so rejuvenated him that his superiors not only welcomed him back into the fold but gave him a coveted promotion as well. Slimfasting gave him a new and youthful lease on a long life.

WHY THIS SLIMFASTING PLAN ERASED POUNDS-INCHES

The law of "compensation" or "atonement" is evident here. While many calories and carbohydrates and fats were taken in on the "odd-numbered days," they were metabolized on the "even-numbered days" when very low calorie-carbohydrate (fat-free) vegetables were eaten. This gave him appetite-satisfaction and weight loss at the same time.

REGULATES METABOLISM, CONTROLS APPETITE

During this Slimfasting program, the digestive tract is rewarded with a physiological rest (on the even-numbered days) which helps regulate metabolism and control appetite. There is a gentle reduction of what is known as the *food-conditioned reflex leucocytosis;* the excitative-appetite processes become reduced. This reduction reaches the cortex of the brain where there is a blocking of the appetite stimuli.

Simultaneously, with the reduction of the secretory and vascular reflexes, there is a mobilization of detoxifying defense mechanisms that are known for neutralizing toxic wastes and dissolving accumulated fat-calories-carbohydrates and then washing them out through the eliminative channels of the body.

There is also a rise in the levels of blood sugar and this helps create a feeling of appetite satisfaction with reduced food intake.

The improved metabolism is then able to use body enzymes (freed from the responsibility of digesting food during a fast day) to break down and help dissolve the subcutaneous deposits in the *adipose* tissues and create slimming and weight loss.

EAT AND REDUCE

When Edgar R. fasted on the even-numbered days, this miraculous internal weight-melting mechanism was put in full gear and weight was washed out of his body. When Edgar R. ate on the odd-numbered days, the "compensation" principle was put into effect. That is, he could eat 1500 calories through sweets and his beer. But they were speedily metabolized on the even-numbered days when he went on an all raw-vegetable program of Slimfasting. So Edgar R. could "eat and reduce" on this simple yet welcome reducing plan. Furthermore, as long as he remained on this easy Slimfasting plan, the weight would stay off *permanently*.

How to Feel Energetic and Healthy During Slimfasting

Before starting any fast of any length, receive approval from your doctor. You should not fast if you have doctor-diagnosed heart trouble, especially a tendency toward thrombosis. Also you should obtain approval of your doctor if you have diagnosed problems of a tumor, bleeding ulcer, active pulmonary disease, diabetes, gout, liver or kidney ailments, cerebral disorders, recent myocardial infarction as well as a blood infection. There are reported healings of such ailments under supervised fasting, but you should discuss this with your physician.

Folks who are able to fast and want to keep feeling energetic and healthy during their program should follow these suggestions:

Keep Warm. While your metabolism is being "readjusted," you should avoid being chilled. Keep yourself warmly dressed. At night, snuggle under warm bedclothes.

Enjoy Moderate Sunbathing. You will find comfort if you enjoy moderate sunbathing. Keep your head covered. Drink lots of liquids to replace those lost during healthy perspiration. Avoid the very hot midday hours, however.

Balance Work with Rest. During your Slimfasting program, keep yourself active but don't overdo it. Avoid strenuous mental or physical work. Be sure to obtain a full eight or ten hours of sleep every night.

Bathe Away Toxic Wastes. Nightly, take comfortably warm baths. Take *short* baths to avoid enervation. About 20 minutes as you wash away toxic wastes with a washcloth would be most helpful.

Water Drinking Is Important. Drinking large amounts of water is important on all Slimfasting programs. This helps your kidneys excrete stored up wastes as well as debris from fatty tissues. Water temperature should be at a comfortable room temperature. NO ice water. NO boiling hot water. If you dislike ordinary tap water because of chemical additives, look into bottled spring water. If possible, avoid distilled water. True, it is pure but it has NO minerals, and, fasting or not, your body needs minerals. You may also enjoy mineral water. Both bottled spring water and mineral water may be found at most health stores, or look in the classified telephone directory under "water" for home deliveries.

Mild Exercise Is Helpful. More calories will be burned up when you exercise. Simple and healthy calorie-burning exercises include walking (try for 60 to 90 minutes a day at a brisk and unhurried pace). Try bicycle riding, golf, bowling. Whittle down your waist by dancing regularly! DO NOT jog or go in for long-distance running since this may be too strenuous for you at this time.

General Guidelines. Avoid sudden movements such as jumping out of bed hurriedly, chasing after a bus or train, running up or down stairs. Prepare yourself *in advance* for the activity and ease gently into it. DO NOT take unprescribed and unsupervised pills or drugs of any kind. DO NOT smoke. DO NOT use any chemical cosmetics (these block skin pores and seal in toxins that need to be eliminated). DO NOT use chemicalized toothpaste or mouthwash. Instead, use a little baking soda on your toothbrush and in a glass of warm water for a refreshing mouthwash.

With periodic Slimfasting, you enable your body's self-healing powers of metabolism and assimilation to perform miracles of reshaping, revitalizing and rejuvenation. You'll also be able to shed pounds and melt inches—quickly and permanently!

IN REVIEW

1. Slimfasting promotes internal cleansing. It creates a form of natural rejuvenation. It is not starvation since you can eat while you Slimfast your way to a healthier body.

2. It's easy to set your goals, then follow the eight starter steps for Slimfasting.

3. Follow the step-by-step guide to Slimfasting from start to slim finish.

4. A simple Slimfasting program trimmed Michael B.'s waistline from 54 to 35 in three short weeks.

5. Edgar R. followed a delicious "odd-even" day Slimfasting program that saved his job, improved his health, erased over 50 pounds.

6. Feel healthy and energetic during your Slimfasting program with the listed suggestions. It makes reducing a sheer joy!

Chapter Three

Easy One Day, Three Day, Weekend Slimfasting to Melt 5-10-15 Stubborn Pounds

A Slimfasting program that can help you melt from 5 to 15 (and more) stubborn pounds calls for enjoying most of your favorite foods but with limits and controls on the intake of two weight-causing compounds: carbohydrates and calories. This Slimfasting program permits you to enjoy most of your favorite meats, fish, poultry, dairy foods but calls for "compensation" whereby you go on a low to very low "carbo-cal" program. This creates a metabolic reaction wherein the stubborn pounds that refuse to be melted can be "loosened" and "broken up" and eliminated within a short span of time, often a few days or a weekend.

Scientific Journals Back Up Her Confidence

A researcher, Helen K., learned about the value of fasting in her reading. A trip to the library opened up a new vista about this modern method of weight loss. She discovered endless amounts of scientific papers, monographs, articles, books, reports authored by specialists in the field on the benefits of controlled fasting for weight loss. With this array of published documents by scientific journals, Helen K. now had all the confidence she needed. She applied the methods based on reports issued by clinicians and she was able to lose weight—and keep it off—and feel satisfied with many of her favorite foods.

HOW WEEKEND SLIMFASTING MELTS STUBBORN POUNDS

Helen K. had gained over 40 pounds after the birth of her three children over a period of seven years. She had gone through the "diet game" as she called it and managed to lose about 25 pounds. But she had 15 stubborn pounds that refused to melt away. Furthermore, Helen K. feared more pounds would be added if she could not adjust her metabolism to help dissolve and cast out the "fat 15" as she called them. She turned to a simple weekend Slimfasting program that called for very low "carbo-cal" intake while she could enjoy her favorite foods. Here is the simple program that helped melt away her "fat 15" stubborn pounds:

SAY "NO" TO "CARBO-CAL" FOODS

Helen K. would say "no" to any foods that contained high amounts of either carbohydrates or calories or both. Instead, she would select lean meats, the white meat of chicken or turkey, lean fish, dairy products made from skim milk, and as much water, herb tea, or a coffee substitute such as Postum that she preferred. She followed this Weekend Slimfasting program for only three days. She weighed herself twice daily. She actually saw the way her "fat 15" stubborn pounds melted away. Once they were gone, Helen K. looked forward to a wonderful life with a new slim-svelte figure. If she ever gained back excess pounds, she would go on a Weekend Slimfasting program and say "no" to "carbo-cal" foods. This let her enjoy most of her favorite foods while she shed pounds and inches.

HOW A "CARBO-CAL SLIMFASTING"
PROGRAM MELTS POUNDS

Two major weight-causing substances are carbohydrates and calories. (See Figure 3-1.) When stored in the body, they turn into fat that adds pounds and inches. During a Slimfasting program that cuts down or eliminates intake of these nutrients, the process of metabolism causes the spontaneous combustion or "heat generation" process whereby sufficient ketone bodies (incompletely burned fat) cause elimination of ketones in amounts sufficient to account for remarkable rates of weight loss.

Such a Slimfasting program permits you to eat your favorite foods but calls for restriction of foods containing sugar and starch in large amounts. The metabolic reaction is swift when "carbo-cal" foods are restricted and the metabolic process calls for self-feeding so that accumulated weight is oxidized and melted away. This can help cast out pound after pound after pound of stubborn fat in a short time.

CALORIE •CARBOHYDRATE CHART

Abbreviations:
A = Average
AS = Average Serving

C = Cup
L = Large

M = Medium
S = Slice

Sm. = Small
Sq. = Square

T = Tablespoon
t = teaspoon

Item	Portion	Calories	Carbohydrate Grams
Almonds	15	100	4
American Cheese	1S	100	Trace
Angel Food Cake	AS	200	32
Apple	M	50	22.6
Apple, dried, cooked without sugar	M	122	31.7
Apple Juice	1C	100	26
Apple Dumpling	1M	300	54
Apple Pie	AS	350	51
Apple Sauce	1/2C	150	26
Apricots, Dried	3M	50	13.8
Apricots with syrup	3M	75	26
Apricots	3M	100	25
Apricot Pie	AS	350	57.7
Asparagus Soup	1C	147	16.6
Bacon	1S	30.5	.16
Banana	1M	100	26
Banana Split	A	400	92.5
Barley	1/4C	150	39
Bass	AS	100	0
Bean Soup	1C	170	22
Beans baked	1/2C	261	47.77
Beans, Kidney	1/2C	81	14.76
Beans, Lima (Baby)	1/2C	94	17.84
Beans, String	1C	44	10.2
Beef Boiled	AS	250	0
Beef Broth	1C	30	3
Beef chopped	AS	100	0
Beef Chuck/ground	AS	363	0
Beef/Round Steak	AS	292.32	0
Beets	1/4C	21	5
Berry Pies	AS	350	56
Biscuits	1Sm.	129	16
Blackberries	1/2C	42.5	9.5
Blueberries	1/2C	42.5	10.5
Bologna	2S	150	2.2
Bouillon cube	1	2	0
Bran Flakes	1/2C	50	14
Bread, white	1S	62	11.6

Figure 3-1

Item	Portion	Calories	Carbohydrate Grams
Broccoli	1C	40	7
Brussels Sprouts	2/3C	36	6
Butter	1Pat	50	Trace
Buttermilk	1C	75	12
Cabbage boiled	1/4C	7	1.5
Cabbage raw	1/4C	4	1
Candy, chocolate	1 oz.	133	17.8
Cantaloupe	1/2	115.5	28.87
Carrots	1/2C	22.5	5
Catsup	1T	25	4.2
Cauliflower	1 1/2C	37	12.5
Celery	1C	15	4
Cherries	1C	133	33.06
Chicken broiled	1/2 Sm.	281.52	0
Chicken roasted	1/2 breast	106.08	0
Chicken Soup	1C	95	8
Chocolate Cake	AS	205	29.12
Chocolate Cookies	6 Sm.	108	17.16
Chocolate Pudding	1/4C	80	62
Chocolate Syrup	1T	46.5	11.9
Cinnamon Toast	1S	200	15.9
Clams	1/2C	83	2.2
Cocoa with milk	1C	212	27
Cocoa powdered	1T	24.9	6.25
Codfish	AS	215	0
Coffee black	1C	2.5	.66
Coffee Cake	AS	90	14
Condensed Milk	1C	980	166
Consomme	1C	21	1.92
Corn	1/4C	42.5	10
Corn Flakes	1/2C	50	11
Corn Oil	1T	125	0
Cottage Cheese	1T	21	.621
Crackers, Soda	6	186	30
Cream	3T	90	1
Cream Cheese	1 oz.	104.72	.588
Cucumber	1A	30	7
Cup Cake	1A	315	48
Doughnut	1A	151	21.7
Duck	AS	109	0
Egg, hard-boiled	1	78	.4
Egg Plant	1/2C	19	4.1
Evaporated Milk	1C	345	.24
Filet of Sole, broiled	AS	105.3	0
Flour, Wheat	1C	409	83.7
Frankfurter	1	182.4	.96
French Dressing	1T	100	3

Figure 3-1 (cont'd.)

Item	Portion	Calories	Carbohydrate Grams
Gelatin/Sweetened	1/2C	140	34
Grapefruit	1/2	50	13
Grapefruit Juice	1/2C	50	12
Grapes	1C	65	15
Haddock, Fried	AS	165	5.8
Halibut, broiled	AS	426	0
Ham	AS	126	0
Hamburger	2 oz.	363	0
Honey	1T	65	17
Honeydew Melon	1/4	33	7.7
Ice Cream	1C	290	29
Jam	1T	55	14
Kale	1/2C	28	4.86
Lamb Chop	1M	260	0
Lamb Roast	AS	119	0
Lemon	1M	20	10.7
Lemon Pie	AS	305	45
Lentils	1/2C	233	41.7
Lettuce	1/4 Head	15	3
Liver, Calf	AS	74	1.7
Lobster, broiled	1	308	.8
Macaroni	1C	190	39
Mackeral, broiled	AS	415.2	0
Meat Loaf	AS	264	11.5
Milk, skim	1C	90	12
Milk, whole	1C	161	12
Muffins	1	125	17
Mushrooms	2/3C	26.6	4
Mustard	1t	3.5	.32
Nectarine	1M	80	21.37
Noodles	1/2C	100	18
Oatmeal	1/2C	65	16
Okra	1/2C	34.2	7.92
Olive Oil	1T	125	0
Olives	3 Sm.	15	Trace
Onion raw	1M	40	10
Onion cooked	3M	180	42
Orange	1M	75	14
Orange Juice	1C	110	26
Oysters, raw	12	104	5
Parmesan Cheese	1T	25	Trace
Parsnips	1M	121	28
Peaches canned	1C	200	52

Figure 3-1 (cont'd.)

Item	Portion	Calories	Carbohydrate Grams
Peaches fresh	1M	35	10
Peach Pie	AS	421	63
Peanut Butter	1T	93	3.12
Peanuts	1/4C	336	11.16
Pears fresh	1 Sm.	100	25
Pears canned	1C	195	50
Pears dried	1/2C	50	13
Peas	1/4C	21.2	3.9
Pecans	1C	740	16
Peppers, green	1M	15	4
Pimento Cheese	1 1/2 oz.	150	2.8
Pineapple, fresh	1S	37.44	9.86
Pineapple, canned	1S	45	12
Pineapple Pie	AS	404	61
Plums, canned	1C	205	53
Plums, fresh	1	25	7
Powdered Sugar	1T	30	8
Pork Chop broiled	1M	101.6	0
Pork Roast	AS	380.1	0
Pork Sausage	2	188	0
Postum, no milk	1C	10	2
Pot Roast	AS	339.3	0
Potato baked	1 Sm.	141	32
Potato boiled	1M	110.2	24.79
Potato Chips	1 Chip	11	1.0
Potato, french fried	10 pieces	155	20
Potato mashed	1/2C	62.5	12.5
Potato Salad	1/2C	99	16.3
Potato Soup	1C	105	12
Potato Sweet	1M	15	4
Prunes	3	52.5	13.5
Prune Juice	1/2C	100	24
Pumpkin Pie	AS	275	32
Radishes	5M	10	1.8
Raisin Pie	AS	325	32.5
Raisins	1/4C	125	128
Raspberries canned	1/2C	50	21.4
Raspberries fresh	1/2C	50	23.5
Rhubarb, stewed	1C	211	54
Roast Beef	AS	261	0
Roquefort Cheese	AS	150	.5
Roquefort Dressing	1T	125	1.2
Round Steak	AS	254	0
Rutabaga	1/2C	35	8.2
Ry-Krisp	5	100	19.2
Salmon, Red	1C	427	0
Sardines	3	233	.45
Sauerkraut	1/2C	27.5	4.5
Scallops, steamed	1C	112	0

Figure 3-1 (cont'd.)

Item	Portion	Calories	Carbohydrate Grams
Shrimp, breaded	1	31.97	4.57
Sirloin Steak	AS	261	0
Sour Cream	1T	30.3	.625
Spaghetti	1C	155	32
Spinach	1/2C	20	3
Squash hubbard	1/2C	36	8.9
Squash summer	1/4C	15	3.5
Strawberries	1C	55	13
Succotash canned	1/2C	89	19.7
Sugar, white	1t	20	6
Swiss Cheese	1S	68	Trace
Tangerine	1L	40	10
Tapioca Pudding	1/2C	100	11.6
Tea plain	1C	2	.4
Tomato	1	40	9
Tuna, cooked	1C	315	0
Turkey	AS	70.4	0
Turnips	1/2C	18	4
Veal Chop	1M	107.6	0
Vegetable Soup	1C	84	8
Watercress	1C	4	.6
Watermelon	1S Sm.	115	27
Wheaties	1/2C	75	12
Whipped Cream	3T	30	Trace
White Fish steamed	AS	275.8	0
Yams	1M	210	48.2

Figure 3-1 (cont'd.)

HOW A THREE DAY "MEAT SLIMFASTING" PROGRAM CREATES NEW SLIMNESS

Husband and wife, George and Eleanor C. loved to eat thick steaks smothered in onions, and often shared the joys of eating thick chops swimming in natural juices. Both of them were 25 pounds overweight. But they refused to give up their love for luscious, juicy, succulent cuts of meat. So they both decided to go on a special three day "Meat Slimfasting" program that let them continue eating their favorite meats but was very low in "carbo-cal" foods. This three day Slimfasting program melted away their 25 overweight pounds and they could continue eating their meats.

Basic Program: George and Eleanor C. selected a variety of different meats to enjoy during their three day Slimfasting program.

They eliminated all high "carbo-cal" foods from their eating program. It was as simple as that and it helped melt away their overweight pounds during one three day weekend!

WHAT A MEAT SLIMFASTING PROGRAM CAN DO TO LOSE POUNDS

The "carbo-cal" content in foods causes weight, not necessarily the fat in meats. "Carbo-cal" causes weight gain by blocking the body's natural metabolism that burns up fat. A Meat Slimfasting Program creates what is known as a *Thermodynamic Combustion Reaction* (TCR) in the system. In the Absence of additional "carbo-cal" elements from foods, the TCR process releases energy into your bloodstream, prompts the stored fat to be melted and washed out of your system. The "villains" are both carbohydrates and calories. When there is a restriction of intake of these "villains" in the body, then the TCR mechanism goes into effect and the process of *autolysis* or "self-loosening" occurs and accumulated "carbo-cal" deposits are cast out of the body.

The luscious taste of favorite meats offers appetite satisfaction; there is a feeling of contentment because the high protein in the meats soothes stomach hunger contractions and eases the gnawing hunger urge. This helps you feel "well fed" while you lose pounds while eating meats.

How Weekend Slimfasting Creates "TCR" Weight Loss

The secret of effectiveness of a weekend Slimfasting program is that in a short time it helps create what is known as *Thermodynamic Combustion Reaction* or TCR. This is the secret principle involved in swift weight loss through a weekend of Slimfasting.

HOW TCR CAUSES WEIGHT LOSS

Pounds and inches are caused by accumulated carohydrates and calories. When these elements are restricted during a weekend Slimfasting, the process of *Thermodynamic Combustion Reaction* can work freely. Weight loss occurs as follows:

The TCR converts accumulated fats into carbohydrates. Metabolically, carbon chain fatty acids stored in adipose (fat) tissue triglycerides are mobilized for use in the appreciable net synthesis of carbohydrate. The TCR breaks down these substances to release glycerol during hydrolysis of triglyceride and create weight loss. This breaks down the triglyceride accumulation and causes their components to be oxidized. This is possible through the Thermodynamic

Combustion Reaction, when your body is spared the task of metabolizing additional "carbo-cal" intake and thus turns "inward" to "feed upon" the accumulated "villains" and thereby help metabolize and dissolve them out of your system. The TCR principle works most effectively when you restrict intake of "carbo-cal" foods so there is little *competition* for your metabolism which can then freely use the TCR process for the oxidizing and evaporation of accumulated elements. It works swiftly during a weekend or during a short period of time with no denial of most of your favorite foods. It is the quick and delicious way to weight loss.

THE 4-DAY 20-POUNDS OFF SLIMFASTING PROGRAM

Blanche E. had an expanding waistline that even a tight girdle failed to conceal. Her face became heavy and a double chin marred what could have been a lovely neck. Her arms and shoulders were heavy. There were times when she had to gasp for breath after climbing a few steps. She looked much older than her 42 years. But try as she would, Blanche could not melt away the aging 20 pounds of overweight. While dieting had helped her lose many pounds and inches, it could not get these last 20 pounds off her body. So it was that she took the advice of friends and set up a planned, "20-pounds off" Slimfasting program during a four-day weekend. Blanche E. confessed that she loved the taste of luscious meats and this was the bane of her overweight. So a Slimfasting program that permitted her to indulge in meats would make her feel "filled up" while she would "slim down." Here is the simple, delicious and effective 4-day 20-pounds off Slimfasting program that did the slimming trick:

BREAKFAST

1/2 grapefruit *or* 8 ounces unsweetened grapefruit juice

2 eggs scrambled or prepared in any desired style

4 slices of lean meat

1 cup herb tea or a coffee substitute such as Postum

LUNCHEON

1/2 grapefruit *or* 8 ounces unsweetened grapefruit juice

Beef or *any* pure meat, either baked, broiled, boiled or fried with any amount of butter sauce and natural meat juice for gravy

All the lettuce or salad you want with apple cider vinegar-oil dressing

1 cup herb tea or a coffee substitute such as Postum

DINNER

1/2 grapefruit *or* 8 ounces unsweetened grapefruit juice

Cold, boiled or baked meat of any desire, sautéed in butter and natural meat juice for gravy

Chopped lettuce with apple cider vinegar-oil dressing

1 cup herb tea or a coffee substitute such as Postum

ENJOY THESE FOODS

Vegetables: Select very low carbo-cal vegetables such as broccoli, spinach, cauliflower, squash, cabbage and eat as much as you want. *Suggestion:* Drain off all liquid from cooked vegetables.

Fats: Use as much butter as you prefer. For salad dressing, use olive oil instead of any other oil since it is very very low in carbo-cal content and offers good taste. The use of margarine is a matter of taste.

How "TCR" Helped Evaporate 20 Pounds in 4 Days

Blanche E. followed this simple 4-day program which let her indulge in her luscious and succulent favorite meats. She weighed herself at the end of the 4th day. With an exclamation of joy, she discovered that she had lost those 20 pounds! When she looked in the mirror, she saw her chin looking firm and youthful with a swan-like neck. Her arms and shoulders looked and felt light. She could walk up and down steps with youthful agility. To crown off the rewards of this tasty Slimfasting program, Blanche E. looked and felt years younger! She felt it was a miracle!

The principle of *Thermodynamic Combustion Reaction* created what Blanche E. considered a miracle in melting away the 20 pounds in so short a time as a *four day weekend!* The TCR went into effect when Blanche E. restricted intake of carbohydrates and calories. There was a slow decrease in the amount of triglycerides. This created the generation of enough ketone bodies that would cause the expulsion of broken down fatty tissues and a corresponding weight loss.

BENEFIT OF A WEEKEND SLIMFASTING PROGRAM

During this short timespan, your body *reuses* the stored up carbo-cal supplies that are causing you overweight. This obviates the need for constant replenishment over this short timespan. By reusing the stored up supplies of carbohydrates and calories through the *Thermodynamic Combustion Reaction* or TCR for a *short* timespan, your body can continue to function healthfully with reduced or controlled intake of carbo-cal elements. You emerge from your Weekend Slimfasting Program with a look and feel of youthful vitality. Weight is lost, inches are slimmed down, and good health is yours again.

HOW TO MELT AWAY INCHES
DURING A 3-DAY SLIMFASTING PROGRAM

Pick any holiday weekend, or it may be any 3-day weekend, or any available 3-day timespan for your simple Slimfasting program. Now follow this simple step-by-step method that will take away inches from your waistline, hips and other body parts!

You Will Need: Natural brown rice (avoid precooked rice which has less texture, more calories and is deficient in important nutrients), a variety of seasonings, soy sauce, available seasonal fruits, Chinese noodles, lean meat, poultry and any low-calorie vegetables.

BREAKFAST

Combine one-half cup cooked brown rice with large amounts of fresh seasonal fruit such as berries, diced cantaloupe, peach or banana slices, citrus fruit sections. *Tip:* Sprinkle with cinnamon for a delicious sweet-satisfaction taste.

LUNCHEON

One cup cooked brown rice
One cup mixed vegetables with Chinese noodles
Use desired seasonings such as soy sauce

DINNER

Low-calorie vegetable dish of brown rice with mushrooms, broccoli, cabbage, stewed tomatoes with desired seasonings
Lean broiled meat (trim off all visible fat) sliced paper thin
Suggestion: In place of beef or veal, use diced or chunked chicken

Slimfasting Benefits: These three meals are filling and satisfying. Fruits offer a delicious sweet taste. Meats offer a feeling of fat satiety with little "hard" fat. The total intake is under 1000 calories for all three meals! The carbohydrate intake is modest, too.

HOW THERMODYNAMIC COMBUSTION REACTION MELTS AWAY INCHES

When you Slimfast on this 3-day program, your metabolism is spared the obligation of a strong protein digesting function because there is minimal fat intake. Instead, the vitamins, minerals and enzymes are given "star priority." They are used by your *Thermodynamic Combustion Reaction* or TCR to shrink the excess subcutaneous fat (located directly beneath skin surface) and this starts the "inch shrink" process that helps create youthful slimness.

TCR then helps oxidize the *muscle-mass* fibers and tissues so that more inches start to come off. During the preceding 3-day Slimfasting program, the large amount of vitamins, minerals and enzymes are used to transform bulging fat cells into tissues that can be used to repair and replenish those that are broken down.

TCR creates this internal environment so that extra fat is actually sucked out from between the muscles and this helps reduce the girth of such problem areas as your stomach, hips, buttocks, shoulders, arms and legs. On such a Slimfasting program, TCR can help melt away unsightly and age-causing inches during a 3-day span.

THE SLIMFASTING JELLY PROGRAM

It is reported[1] that Europeans use a Slimfasting jelly program that melts away stubborn pounds in a matter of days. It's called the *gel de froment,* a bland porridge jelly made of wheat flakes dissolved in freshly boiled water.

How to Take It: Europeans drink four plates of this *gel de froment* daily, with fresh lemon, grapefruit or orange juice to complete the Slimfasting program. That's all there is to it.

Added Flavor: For added flavor, use vegetable broth instead of water. Add a large spoonful of aromatic herbs.

Fast Weight Loss: This Slimfasting jelly program offers speedy weight loss—*a reported two pounds a day.* This may be too quick for some folks but it's a popular Slimfasting program in Europe.

Wheat flakes or wheat germ are available in most supermarkets and in health stores.

---

[1] Courtesy *Parker Natural Health Bulletin,* West Nyack, New York 10994. Vol. 5, No. 22, October 22, 1975. Available by subscription.

Benefits: The wheat flakes offer a feeling of appetite satisfaction and fullness. Brimming with vitamins, minerals, grain protein, these nutrients are used by the enzymes in the fresh fruit juice to help dissolve accumulated fat and reduce inches.

HOW SLIMFASTING SLIMS DOWN INCHES

Weight is caused by the accumulation of fat interspersed with the muscle mass in your body. (This can be seen in butcher shop beef where meat is sliced against the grain; fat is between fibers and tissues. This is called "marbleized meat" because it looks like the markings in marble.)

When the fat is removed from between the muscle fibers and tissues, then the bulk starts to become reduced. The mass shrinks in external dimensions.

During the Slimfasting program using the above European *gel de froment,* the areas of the body that bulge will start to shrink as the fat is removed from between muscle fibers and tissues. As more fat is pulled out from the muscle area, the inches around the waist, buttocks, thighs, legs, and other noticeable areas, also start to be reduced and come down. This creates the youthful slimness, the svelte shape, the romantic silhouette figure that is symbolic of good health and attractive weight.

THE "BA" WAY TO NATURAL WEIGHT LOSS[2]

It is reported that "Behavioral Approach" is a new and simple— but very effective way to lose weight. During *any* Slimfasting program, you may still have a desire to overeat. Try the BA way that calls for understanding *what* you eat, *when* and *where* you eat it and *how much.* These factors have been grouped under what is referred to as "behavioral approach" or a "situational control" whereby you recognize that overeating is controlled not solely by yourself, but by others and by the places in which you eat and live.

Examples: You have a tendency to overeat when you watch television, especially when you are tempted by commercials selling super-delicious cakes. Therefore, prepare yourself *in advance* by keeping such fattening foods as potato chips and other goodies out of reach of your TV set. A good BA attitude is *not* to have such fattening foods in your house in the first place. Avoid temptation and you avoid overeating.

---

[2]Courtesy *Parker Natural Health Bulletin,* West Nyack, New York 10994. Vol. 5, No. 26, December 22, 1975. Available by subscription.

How to Use Behavioral Approach
Methods with Slimfasting

Combine BA with Slimfasting for quick pound and inch loss, in these ways:

1. Eat in one room only; do not associate eating with any other part of the house, especially a spot close to the TV set. The reason for this is that you have learned to be hungry in places where you have eaten and when doing things (such as watching TV) that have been paired with eating.

2. Do grocery shopping *after* you have eaten. Take along only enough money for what you have sensibly planned to buy. Prepare a shopping list that includes healthful, nutritious and non-fattening foods *only*. Don't cheat! You'll only fool yourself.

3. Others in your family can help by telling you if you are overeating; they can compliment you when you are not.

4. Select a Slimfasting program and stick to it. Do not skip any meals. This simply makes you over-hungry when you do eat.

5. Eat slowly. It takes about 20 minutes for your brain to get the message that enough has been eaten. If you eat more slowly, the message will get there before you have eaten all you might otherwise stuff yourself with.

6. Eat only what your Slimfasting program suggests. Also, plan your Slimfasting meals ahead. Avoid spontaneous or careless eating.

7. Eat only one forkful at a time. Keep telling yourself that you do not have to rush with your meal. Slow down. Enjoy your food. You will feel fuller even though you have eaten less.

8. Don't feel ashamed about leaving something on your plate. This shows *you* have control over the food—not the food over you.

With this new method of "Behavioral Approach" combined with Slimfasting, you can continue enjoying most of your favorite foods while you lose pounds and inches.

THE SLIMFASTING "DEAMOF" PROGRAM[3]
FOR FAST WEIGHT LOSS

A simple Slimfasting program is the "Deamof "Diet that can be followed for two, three or four days to help melt up to 10 pounds that might otherwise cling like "glue."

Deamof stands for "Don't eat anything made of flour." This includes bread, toast, biscuits, muffins, corn bread, cookies, cakes, gravies, sauces, pancakes, waffles, pies, puddings, popovers, prepared breakfast foods, spaghetti, macaroni, ravioli, noodles, etc.

What Can You Eat? Lots of fresh fruits and vegetables, lean meats, poultry, raw and cooked salads, lean fish, beans, peas, nuts, seeds, eggs (three per week), dairy products made from skim milk.

How Slimfasting Works: The *Deamof* program is very low in carbohydrates and calories. Therefore, your body's *Thermodynamic Combustion Reaction* is able to turn *inward* to your adipose cells and dissolve the stored up carbo-cal weight-causing elements and help wash them out of your system. It is a tasty way to better health through youthful slimness.

12 WAYS TO BOOST YOUR THERMODYNAMIC
COMBUSTION REACTION POWERS

For more effective results during any Slimfasting program, you need to boost and energize your body's built-in *Thermodynamic Combustion Reaction* powers. The more effective your TCR, the more effective your melting of pounds and inches. Here are 12 ways to alert-activate-amplify your TCR powers:

1. During Slimfasting, drink at least two quarts of water every day.
2. Keep active through moderate exercise such as walking, bowling, moderate swimming, bicycle riding.
3. Restrict the use of any pills or medication except with your doctor's approval and guidance.
4. Keep your body warm. Avoid being chilled.
5. As often as possible, get out into the fresh air.
6. If possible, try to take occasional naps in the outdoors, in the shade.

[3]Courtesy *Parker Natural Health Bulletin,* West Nyack, New York 10994. Vol. 6, No. 11, May 24, 1976. Available by subscription.

7. Alert your metabolism through controlled sunbathing. A 30 minute exposure before 11:00 A.M., and another one after 2:00 P.M. would be helpful. That is, 30 minutes in the morning and 30 minutes in the late afternoon. Keep your head covered. Avoid sunburning.

8. Avoid dehydration by drinking healthful beverages. Use herb teas, coffee substitutes such as Postum. You may want to try non-calorie soft drinks if you are very thirsty, although these may contain caffeine and carbonic acid which may disturb your TCR balance.

9. Avoid tobacco in all its forms.

10. Avoid alcoholic beverages in all their forms.

11. Several times daily, take a tepid shower or bath. During your Slimfasting program, the TCR process is dissolving wastes and toxic accumulations which have to be cast out through your billions of skin pores. A bath opens your pores so the TCR process can more effectively eliminate these wastes and create better internal health. *Tip:* Invigorate the TCR process by using a rough wash cloth to rub all over your skin during a bath.

12. Avoid any sudden motions. The TCR process is creating many internal adjustments so avoid jerky, sudden, spasmodic movements as these may make you dizzy. Emotionally and physically prepare for whatever you have in mind. In brief, don't surprise your body!

Also avoid extremes of hot and cold in baths or foods or in going from one room to the other. With these easy-to-follow suggestions, you should be able to help your body unlock the mechanism and enable your metabolism to use the *Thermodynamic Combustion Reaction* to help "uproot" stubborn carbo-cal-fat combinations and dissolve them. This will enable you to use a Slimfasting program that will melt 5-10-15 (or more) stubborn pounds and inches during one, two, three or four days. It's the natural way to Slimfast your way to better health.

SUMMARY

1. Lose weight and inches within a few days with easy-to-follow Slimfasting programs.

2. Helen K. used an easy Slimfasting program that helped her melt 15 stubborn pounds during one weekend.

3. George and Eleanor C. loved the juicy taste of succulent meats. They had (each) 25 overweight pounds that they wanted to lose in three days without giving up beloved meats. They lost their overweight on a delicious "Meat Slimfasting" program for just three days.

4. Slimfasting creates a *Thermodynamic Combustion Reaction* or TCR that attacks the body's stored up carbo-cal-fat reserves and thereby creates easy and fast slimming.

5. Blanche E. used a simple 4-day 20-pounds off Slimfasting program that not only slimmed down her chin, arms and shoulders, but took off pounds and inches elsewhere. The TCR process made her youthfully slim in a short time.

6. Try a simple 3-day Slimfasting program as outlined to effectively use the TCR process for pounds-inches slimming.

7. Europeans reportedly lose pounds in a few days with the Slimfasting jelly program. Fills you up while it slims you down.

8. Boost the *Thermodynamic Combustion Reaction* process with Behavioral Approach methods in just eight easy steps.

9. The Slimfasting "Deamof" Program can melt up to 10 "glue-like" pounds in a few days . . . while you continue to eat almost all of your favorite foods.

10. Boost your TCR powers with the easy 12 steps as outlined.

Chapter Four

How to Use Raw Juice Fasting
to Win the Battle of the Bulge

A raw juice fasting program offers you two basic benefits: (1) It will help create easy slimming with reduction of unsightly bulges and (2) It will give you a feeling of appetite satisfaction with a cheerful disposition. When you go on a raw juice fast, the nutrients in the fruits and vegetables help rebuild your billions of body cells and tissues to promote youthful health.

SLIMS BULGES, CREATES REJUVENATION

During a raw juice fast, the process of *autolysis* or self-digestion causes the process of burning up accumulated wastes and tissues. The vitamins, minerals, and enzymes in raw juices will activate your eliminative process to wash out these accumulated wastes. This helps your body "feed upon itself " and then cast out decaying substances that may be responsible for ill health and unsightly bulges. When the raw juices wash out these accumulations, there is an internal cleansing and a form of rejuvenation. A raw juice fast then causes the body's supply of proteins to create new cells and tissues and therefore the process of internal (and subsequently external) rejuvenation is underway. In effect, a raw juice fast is slimming as well as youthifying!

Feel Energetic During a Raw Juice Fast

Raw juices are prime sources of *natural* sugar. It is this *natural* sweet that helps protect against a reaction of hypoglycemia (low blood sugar) that often turns a dieter into a grouch. During a raw juice fast, the natural sugars of the fruits are taken up by the endocrine system to create a response from certain cells in the pancreas (a large, long gland located behind the lower part of the stomach) to secrete a hormone called insulin into the bloodstream.

Insulin enables your body to metabolize blood sugar, that is, to provide energy. During a raw juice fast, the amount of insulin secreted by the *islets of Langerhans* (cells in the pancreas) will be just enough to burn off the excess sugar in the bloodstream, maintaining the blood sugar at a normal level. This is usually between 60 and 100 milligrams of sugar for every 100 cubic centimeters of blood.

It is this stabilized blood sugar level created by the amount of healthy natural sugar in raw fruit and, to some degree, vegetable juices that will sweeten your disposition and make you feel energetic and cheerful during your Slimfasting program.

In preparing for your Raw Juice Slimfasting program, here is a step-by-step program.

DO-IT-YOURSELF "BULGES OFF" RAW JUICE SLIMFASTING PROGRAM

1. Plan ahead for your Raw Juice Slimfasting program. Decide the amount of days for the program. Arrange to have a supply of fresh fruits and vegetables in your refrigerator. You may also need to buy new *fresh* plant foods during the duration of your fast. Prepare for this.

2. Two days *before* your scheduled Raw Juice Slimfasting, prepare your digestive system by eating nothing but any available fruits and vegetables. Chew thoroughly. Obtain adequate nightly rest.

3. On the first and subsequent days of your Raw Juice Slimfasting program, follow this tasty schedule:

BEFORE BREAKFAST: Drink a cup of herb tea with a squeeze of fresh lemon juice and a bit of honey.

BREAKFAST: Drink one glass of equal amounts of any desired raw fruit or vegetable juice with freshly poured cold water.

MID-MORNING: Drink one glass of any desired raw fruit or vegetable juice.

LUNCHEON: Drink two glasses of any desired raw fruit or vegetable juice.

MID-AFTERNOON: Prepare a cup of vegetable broth made of favorite freshly washed vegetables that have been cooked to a "juice-like" consistency and then strained.

DINNER: Drink two glasses of any desired raw fruit or vegetable juice.

NIGHT CAP: Drink one cup of vegetable broth.

Suggestions: Because of the wide variety of different fruits and vegetables available, you should feel free to diversify and enjoy different juices. Combine different fruit juices as a "cocktail" if desired. Combine different vegetable juices as a "tonic" for zesty taste. Do *not* combine fruit and vegetable juices. The cellular slimming reaction may become weakened since the strong elements of natural sugar in the fruit become diluted if the "scrubbing" fiber of the vegetables is added. Drink fruit juices at separate intervals from vegetable juices for more effective Slimfasting.

Keep Active, Clean, Alert. As you juice fast, keep yourself active. Take regular walks. Do mild housework. Go about your daily tasks. Nightly, take a comfortably warm bath or shower. Keep your mind alert by taking an interest in social activities and other events. Daily, weigh yourself. Daily, tape measure your bulges to see how weight loss is helping to slim down unsightly bulges and inches.

HOW TO BREAK YOUR
RAW JUICE SLIMFASTING PROGRAM

It is essential to break your fast properly. When you have completed your scheduled amount of "pounds and inches off" and want to resume your regular plan, follow these rules:

First Day after Fast: Start by eating a few freshly washed *whole apples* in the morning to be followed by one or two cups of herb tea with lemon juice and honey. At noontime, enjoy a *small* bowl of freshly washed *raw* vegetables together with a glass of juice and, if desired, a cup of broth. At dinnertime, have another plate of *raw* vegetables that you chew very slowly and thoroughly.

Second Day after Fast: Soak sun-dried figs or prunes (or combinations) in slightly boiled water. When cool, eat the figs or prunes together with the water. For lunch, a bowl of fresh vegetables. For dinner, a bowl of fresh vegetable soup. You may eat several apples in between meals and enjoy fresh juice whenever desired.

Third Day after Fast: Have the same sun-dried figs or prunes with the water. Have one cup of yogurt. A handful of raw seeds or nuts completes the breakfast. For lunch, have a larger raw salad and add a baked or boiled potato with a dab of oil. For dinner, have one slice of whole grain bread with a bit of oil or butter. Add a slice of natural, non-processed cheese or tablespoon of fat-free cottage cheese, if desired. Have a bowl of vegetable soup.

Fourth Day after Fast: Begin to eat your regular meals but avoid so-called junk food which consists of refined and bleached flour products. Plan to eat as many healthful and natural foods as possible for better health and a slimmer figure.

The basic rules for breaking your Raw Juice Slimfasting program are these:

1. Take care to avoid overeating!
2. All foods should be eaten slowly and very thoroughly chewed!
3. Plan for at least four days of a gradual transition before you begin a normal and healthful eating plan!

RAW JUICES—HOW TO MAKE THEM AND HOW TO USE THEM

1. *Prepare Your Own Juices.* Break down and cleanse accumulated cells and tissues with fresh juices that are free of chemical additives. You can do this by using fresh raw fruits and vegetables from a reputable health store or organic food outlet. If unavailable, then purchase plant foods at your local market and wash them thoroughly under cold water.

2. *Use a Juicer.* Health stores as well as the housewares section of larger department stores sell an electric centrifugal juicer. You may want to have a hydraulic press-type juicer which is also available. It is a lifetime investment for better health.

3. *Wash, Squeeze, Drink.* Freshly wash all plant foods before using. Cut up into smaller pieces. Then put through your juicer until the liquid is squeezed out. (The pulp may also be used as part of your vegetable broth or soup.) Slowly sip the juice. Enjoy its taste. Let the velvety smooth liquid slide down your throat as you feel the elixir of nature create a good feeling throughout your system.

4. *If You Must Store Juices.* For more effective use, juices should be consumed speedily after being prepared. But if you must store, then place the juice in a freshly washed glass jar. Seal tightly. Keep refrigerated. Plan to use as soon after refrigeration as possible.

5. *When to Combine and Not Combine.* You may combine a variety of different fruit OR vegetable juices for various taste thrills. But you should NOT combine fruit and vegetable juices. Never mix them together. *Reason:* When fruit and vegetable juices are combined, there is a slowdown of digestion and assimilation and the reducing process appears to be impaired.

THE FRESH FRUIT FASTING "FFF" WAY TO A SLIM SHAPE

Fresh fruit juices as part of a Slimfasting program will create these miracles of reducing:

1. Fruit juices help replace the need for fat or carbohydrate and have a sparing effect on protein which can then be

　　　freely used by the body for the loosening and metabolizing of accumulated fat-causing elements.

2.　Fruit juices help stimulate gastric secretion and motility and increase the flow of bile so that wastes can be more easily removed from the body.

3.　Fruit juices appear to soothe the hypothalamus (segment of the brain that controls appetite) so there is less of an urge to raid the refrigerator or fall victim to compulsive overeating.

4.　Fruit juices tend to promote better retention of nitrogen, phosphorus, calcium and other elements important for rebuilding new cells and tissues. This is a rejuvenating reaction after the old cells and tissues have been washed out of the system.

5.　Fruit juices are prime sources of needed vitamins, minerals and *natural sugars* that help guard against "cranky" or "grouchy" feelings during dieting. Comparably low in calories, they are deliciously slimming. (See Figure 4-1.)

6.　Fruit juices contain a strange factor which tends to stimulate the micro-electric tension in the tissues. This enables the cells to absorb nutrients directly from the bloodstream and successfully cast out fat-causing metabolic wastes from the adipose tissues. This is the key to the "bulges off" benefit of raw juices.

7.　Nearly 100% of all vital nutritive substances in fruit juices are assimilated directly from the stomach into the bloodstream. There is almost *no* strain on the digestive system. This makes raw juice fasting a comfortable way to melt away bulges and pounds and slim down inches.

A tasty and easy-to-follow FFF or Fresh Fruit Fasting program can help take off pounds and add youthful years to your lifespan.

How a Simple "FFF" Program
Sweetened and Slimmed a Stubborn Overweight

Susan M. was a terror whenever she went on a reducing program. She was grouchy. She would snap upon the slightest provocation. She was miserable to live with and felt miserable herself. On most of her diets, she was denied sugar in any form. This was severe. Because she erroneously denied herself fruits, she developed hypoglycemia or low blood sugar and this created nervous reactions that made her a horror to live with.

Susan M. had 31 overweight pounds. They clung stubbornly

NUTRIENTS IN FRUIT JUICES

(About 4 ounces)

Juice	Calories	Sugar	Potassium	Vitamin A	Vitamin C
		grams	mg.	I.U.	mg.
Acerola juice	23	4.8	–	–	1,600
Apple juice	87	22.0	187	–	2
Apricot juice	49	11.7	3	950	3
Apricot nectar	57	14.6	151	950	6
Blackberry juice	37	7.8	170	–	10
Blueberry juice	54	13.7	111	–	–
Cranberry juice	65	16.5	10	trace	40*
Currant juice	55	13.7	–	–	162
Grapefruit juice	30	7.6	144	–	30
Sugar added	70	17.8	135	–	30
Frozen, diluted	41	9.8	170	10	39
Grape juice	119	29.9	209	–	trace
Guava juice	86	23.9	–	–	100
Lemon juice	23	7.6	141	20	44
Frozen, diluted	44	11.4	16	–	7
Lime juice	4	1.3	16	2	3
Loganberry juice	50	12.4	–	–	–
Orange juice	48	11.2	199	200	40
Frozen. diluted	45	10.7	186	200	45
Papaya juice	60	15.1	–	2,500	51
Peach nectar	48	12.4	78	430	trace
Pear nectar	52	13.2	39	trace	trace
Pineapple juice	55	25.6	284	95	17
Frozen, diluted	52	12.8	136	10	12
Prune juice	77	19.0	235	high	2
Raspberry juice	49	12.8	–	120	18
Sauerkraut juice	10	0.7	none**	–	18
Tangelo juice	41	9.7	–	–	27
Tangerine juice	43	10.2	178	420	22
Frozen, diluted	46	10.8	174	410	27
Tomato juice	19	4.3	227	800	16

*Vitamin C is usually added to bottled cranberry juice.

**Sauerkraut has no potassium and 787 milligrams of sodium—almost 2 percent of the drink. Obviously not a beverage for someone wishing to avoid salt, but a very good reducing beverage. Almost no sugar.

Figure 4-1

because she could never finish a diet since it made her so grumpy. So she quit before these bulges could be disposed of.

One day Susan M. learned she had a dieting choice: Undergo rigid reducing, with a "witch-like temper" that drove everyone (including herself) up against the wall, *or* try a "bulges off" program that would feed her bloodstream *natural fructose* that was nerve-soothing and low in calories. This would be sweet to the taste and disposition. So it was that she discovered the power of the simple FFF program or Fresh Fruit Fasting with the use of *naturally sweet* juices. These fresh juices sent a stream of important fructose to the blood and glands to help soothe her nerves. The natural sugar was metabolized to settle the nervous system and thereby was not used for extensive calorie buildup.

INCHES SHRINK, POUNDS MELT, TEMPER STAYS EVEN

Susan M. prepared herself for a simple four day FFF Slim-fasting program. She acquired a wide variety of different seasonal fresh raw fruits and a juicer. Every day, she prepared her own juices which she enjoyed. Slowly, as the days went on, she saw her inches shrink when she tape-measured herself. Each time she weighed herself, she saw how the pounds had melted. By the end of the fourth day, she had managed to lose three inches from her once-bulging midriff. She had also shed some 25 pounds. But more exciting was her emotional outlook. She was cheerful, happy, energetic, even-tempered throughout the entire tasty "FFF" Slimfasting program. Susan M. had discovered an enjoyable slimming program. She actually loved every bit of it! Now, once a month, she follows this easy FFF Slimfasting program. Her midriff is a neat 29. Her weight is a slim 120. Susan M. is a happy, slim person again.

The reason is that the *natural fruit sugar* in the raw juices helped stabilize her blood sugar level. Her pancreas could use this sugar to create a healthy level of blood sugar and she was calm, delightful to be with, and a happy person. Fresh fruit fasting had transformed her into a slim and healthy person.

THE VEGETABLE JUICE FASTING "VJF" WAY TO YOUTHFUL SLENDERNESS

Fresh vegetable juices offer a unique opportunity for helping to achieve youthful slenderness while building, restoring, and recapturing youthful health at the same time. Here is what fresh vegetable juices can do to help you become rejuvenated:

1. Vegetable juices provide an alkaline surplus in the digestive system which is essential for normalizing the acid-alkaline ratio in the bloodstream and tissues. Much overweight as well as aging can be traced to over-acidity which "clogs" the system with pound-adding debris. Vegetable juices help correct this condition.

2. Vegetable juices offer a treasure of easily-assimilable minerals that help balance amounts in billions of body cells and tissues. This corrects the problem of reduced oxygenation which is a cause of cell-tissue degeneration and weight increase.

3. Vegetable juices contain "plant hormones" which are used by the pancreatic cells *(islets of Langerhans)* to secrete more insulin, which can then metabolize sugar and thereby cause a corresponding weight loss through this oxidation.

4. Vegetable juices contain trace elements in their rich colors which are used by the metabolism to boost the production of red blood corpuscles, stimulate the processes of digestion and assimilation so that "burning" of pound-causing elements is normalized. This helps the body "use up" and "cast out" accumulated weighty substances.

5. Vegetable juices are prime sources of enzymes which prompt the body's hydrochloric acid (digestive substances) to boost metabolism, which helps burn excess fatty substances. This accelerates their removal from the body and a drop in weight.

6. Vegetable juices create a normalizing and stabilizing reaction upon most of the body's physiological and neurological functions. They help soothe the nervous system, improve the thinking, alert the glandular-hormonal networks and wash and rejuvenate the billions of body cells and tissues. This helps promote better assimilation. The process of *autolysis* or "self-loosening" occurs and weighty substances are then cast out of the body. This creates healthful weight loss.

Fresh, raw vegetables prepared in juice form are "slimming tonics" that remake the body and keep it trim and youthful at the same time.

How a "VJF" Slimfasting Plan
Offered Swift Freedom from Fat Bulges

Philip S. looked much older than his 40-plus years. He liked to eat lots of foods, and he had unsightly bulges around his waist (he was ashamed of having people call it a paunch!). Philip S. was already getting so heavy on his chest, with sagging pectorals, that he rarely removed his jacket in the office. He found it difficult to control his appetite. Even when he did try reducing plans, it took so long for the pounds to come off that he lost patience and went back to his regular eating habits—and more pounds.

"VJF" OFFERS SWIFT WEIGHT LOSS

Philip S. wanted to slim down on a program that was fast, uncomplicated and easy. So it was that he turned to the Vegetable Juice Fasting program. It was VJF that did what he wanted.

Simple Schedule: On the first two days of every week, Philip S. would go on a VJF program. He would drink an assortment of different vegetable juices. He would drink them "straight" or combined. He discovered that his "wild appetite" was now tamed. He felt satisfied with a reduced intake of food for the remaining five days of the week.

Results Are Swift. More important, Philip S. saw that "VJF" had rescued him. His "paunch" was shrinking. His belt was being taken in. The heavy, fatty chest deposits started to firm up and flatten out into lean hardness. By the end of the fourth week of just two-days-per-week of the VJF program, Philip S. saw his waistline at a neat 34. His weight was a slim 169. It all happened in a short time.

Easy, Satisfying, Comfortable. The "VJF" Slimfasting program was easy for Philip S. It is satisfying because if offers no distress. It is comfortable because it offers no stomach rumbles, no nervous disorders. Now with so many pounds off and bulges away, he looks much younger. His firm, lean body makes him feel as vibrant, alive and alert as during his college freshman year!

SECRET OF SWIFT WEIGHT LOSS
WITH VEGETABLE JUICE FAST

During the juicing of raw vegetables, all stringy fibers are removed. True, the raw pulp is important. It acts as a "broom" during the peristaltic activity of the intestines. But in severe overweight cases, the pulp slows up the swiftness of assimilation of the juices. Ordinarily, raw vegetables will require several hours of digestive activity. It detracts and slows up normal digestive activity. A "VJF" program relieves the digestive system of the burden of attacking strong, tough woody pulp. Thus spared this burden, the digestive system can now turn toward metabolizing accumulated fats and create swifter weight loss. Raw vegetable juices are speedily assimilated into the system to create this combustion action.

HOW A "GREEN JUICE DRINK" UNLOCKS AND DISPERSES STUBBORN WEIGHT

Laura Y. considered herself a "hopeless" overweight because she was told her weight was "locked" into her system. She had tried a variety of different reducing plans which offered her some weight loss but she still had more than 10 pounds of "stubborn" weight that gave her a bulge around the waist and the threat of a double chin. She not only looked older than she was, she felt it!

"GREEN JUICE DRINK" BREAKS UP FAT

Seeking an easy pound-melting method, Laura Y. turned to the "Green Juice Drink." Her Slimfasting program is simple. One day each week (she prefers Wednesday) she goes on a VJF Slimfasting program. She drinks a freshly prepared Green Juice, three times daily. She takes no other food during that day of the week. After three such Wednesday fastings on the Green Juice Drink, Laura Y. noticed that her waistline was shrinking. She weighed herself. She had lost 8 pounds! By the time her fourth Wednesday came around, she had shed the total 10 pounds and her waistline was very trim and slim. Now, to *maintain* her weight and to protect against regaining the "stubborn" pounds, she devotes every Wednesday to the easy VJF program—three 8 ounce glasses of the miraculous weight-dispersing "Green Juice Drink."

HOW TO MAKE "GREEN JUICE DRINK"

Select any seasonally available green leafy vegetables. These could be lettuce, swiss chard, turnip tops, radish tops, cabbage, celery, mustard greens, sorrel, collards, etc. You may also include carrots, cucumbers, and beets for a bit of added color, but keep these to a minimum. It is important to use *green leafy vegetables*.

Put all of these vegetables into your juicer and squeeze or extract until you have one 8 ounce glass of the green liquid. This is your "Green Juice Drink."

Drink it *slowly*. Salivate *thoroughly*. Enjoy it *fully*.

These actions favor better assimilation and greater effectiveness.

HOW "GREEN JUICE DRINK" CREATES SWIFT WEIGHT LOSS

Green leafy vegetables are grown above the ground, close to the soil. The roots of the vegetables take up a treasure of vitamins, minerals, enzymes from the rich soil. These elements are transported into the "veins" of the leaves. You can see these elements when you hold up a leaf to the light. The thick "veins" of the green leaves are throbbing and pulsating with the rich life's blood of the elements.

When you juice the green leaves, you create a process of *trituration*. This process pulverizes the leaves, grinds open the "veins" and removes the thick source of life for the plant. Locked within are more than just vitamins and minerals, but powerful enzymes that act as miniature "atoms" whereby they can "split open" clumps of digestive fat and accumulated fatty clumps. A "Green Juice Drink" is a powerhouse of these fat-destroying "atoms" created by Nature. They act swiftly. Within 15 minutes after being consumed, they immediately go to work to attack "bulges" and "lumps" as well as "inches" and "pounds" of excess overweight. They "break up" and "disperse" these "targets" and stimulate the eliminative process to cast them out of the system. This "miracle" occurs within a short space of time. If you drink three 8 ounce glasses of this Green Juice, you will be giving your body the working materials needed to "split up" the bulges and help keep you slim—in a short time!

RAW JUICES VS. RAW VEGETABLES

Raw juices from which the pulp has been extracted spare the digestive organs so they can devote full attention to the task of metabolism. Furthermore, the raw juices are prime sources of the fat-destroying "atoms" that might otherwise remain sealed within the leaves. Raw vegetables are important and do require thorough chewing, thorough salivation for digestion and release of the enzymes. For many overweights, this is improperly done. Since overweights already have an overburdened digestive system, it is important to use foods that relieve the burdens. Such foods are raw plant juices. They offer speedy combustion with little digestive efforts and are important for those who seek (and need) swift weight loss.

RAW JUICE FASTING: KEY TO SWIFT
SLIMMING, REFRESHING REJUVENATION

Raw juice fasting offers a double-barreled benefit. It will give a physiological rest to the digestive, assimilative and protective body organs so that the process of metabolism and *autolysis* can create swift slimming through self-digestion. The second benefit: Raw juices help wash away accumulated sludge, debris and waste from the billions of body cells and help create the process of tissue regeneration. This stimulates all body and mind functions and thereby opens the doorway to refreshing rejuvenation.

Slimfasting with raw fruit or vegetable juices offers new hope for a slim youthful life!

HIGHLIGHTS

1. Raw juices create swift *autolysis* (self-digestion) because they require almost no digestion and are speedily assimilated.

2. Try Raw Juice Slimfasting for "bulges-off" within a short space of time. Follow the clearly outlined step-by-step program that shows you how to Slimfast easily *before, during,* and *after.*

3. A tasty FFF or fresh fruit fasting program offers swift weight loss, a cheerful disposition, freedom from hunger pangs.

4. Susan M. used a simple FFF Slimfasting program that made her laugh her way to weight loss.

5. A delicious VJF or vegetable juice fasting program creates an alkaline reaction as well as glandular correction so that weight loss is simple and swift.

6. Philip S. used a simple VJF Slimfasting program that gave him swift freedom from fat bulges. Pounds melted quickly. Rejuvenation was a "fringe benefit" for his Slimfasting.

7. Laura Y. solved her "hopeless" overweight with a fat-dispersing Green Juice Drink taken three times daily during *one* day per week only!

Chapter Five

How a Raw Fruit Fast ("RFF")
Creates Cell-Slimming
for Swift Weight Loss

Fresh raw fruits eaten during a special fasting program can transform your digestive system into an all-natural gigantic cell-slimming engine that will create swift weight loss without any feeling of hunger or discomfort.

"RFF" CREATES INTERNAL COMBUSTION CELL-SLIMMING

A raw fruit fast or RFF creates a form of internal combustion within the digestive system which then slims down the cells for overnight weight loss. Basically, when your body has accumulated an excess amount of sugar and starch, it becomes transformed into fat through your metabolism and stored in cells designed to act as living silos. These are your *adipose storage cells.* The more stored up fat you have in these adipose cells, the more weight you have. To lose weight, you need to alert your metabolism to pierce the membrane of these adipose cells, then dissolve the accumulated fat and wash it out of your system. This is done through a unique and tasty Slimfasting program that calls for going on a *raw fruit fast.* Elements in fresh raw fruits will stimulate your metabolism to create a form of "internal combustion" that will "burn" through the membranes of your adipose storage cells and wash out the fat. This creates a natural, simple and speedy cell-slimming that takes pounds out of your body.

STIMULATES CELL-SLIMMING METABOLISM

A Slimfasting program, during which a wide variety of raw fruits are chewed thoroughly and swallowed with pleasure, creates a unique form of cell-slimming metabolism.

When your digestive system is given nothing but raw fruits, it creates increased micro-electric tension that boosts cell respiration, stimulates cell metabolism, and increases the powers of cell cleansing. This metabolic reaction is then able to enter the membrane of the adipose cells and start to "burn up" the accumulated fat within the *cytoplasm* (body of the cell which stores much fat).

The RFF Slimfasting program then triggers off your metabolism to "burn up" fat storage in the *mitochondria* (power centers within the cell). The RFF will then promote the internal combustion or "burning reaction" in the *ribosomes* (generating stations within the cell membrane). These activities occur within a short time in your millions of adipose cells during an RFF Slimfasting program. When the fat is oxidized and washed out of your system through this process, pounds and inches (as well as bulges) are actually melted right out of your body within a short space of time.

Simple, everyday fresh fruit can create this miracle weight loss within your system during a Slimfasting program of a few days.

RAW FRUIT: ALL-NATURAL REDUCING PILL

Fresh raw fruit can act as an all-natural reducing pill. Fruit is a prime source of an assortment of vitamins, minerals, enzymes, protein, together with unidentified factors that alert and trigger your metabolic system to create the fat-burning combustion that helps pierce and enter the adipose cells and create swift weight loss. (See Figure 5-1.)

"RFF" OFFERS CHEWING SATISFACTION

You can chew your way to weight loss with fresh raw fruit as natural reducing pills. Most fruits need to be thoroughly chewed. You therefore satisfy your chewing urge while at the same time you alert your digestive system to issue forth a supply of enzymes, and these protein-like digestive substances have the power to dissolve strong, stubborn fat accumulations in your cells and promote weight loss. All the while, chewing gives you an important feeling of satisfaction while you lose weight.

"RFF" NOURISHES WHILE IT SLIMS YOU DOWN

Many folks complain that conventional diets deny them important nutrients. For these folks, a nourishing RFF fast is beneficial because it offers a treasure of essential nutrients while it creates Slimfasting. One pound of fruit (see chart in this chapter) offers a variety of vitamins, minerals as well as protein and other essential elements. They nourish your body while they slim you down.

EDIBLE PORTION OF NUTRIENTS IN ONE POUND OF FRUITS

Fruit	Calories	Protein Grams	Carbohydrates mg.	Calcium mg.	Phosphorus mg.	Iron mg.	Sodium mg.	Potassium mg.	Vitamin A I.U.	Thiamine mg.	Riboflavin mg.	Niacin mg.	Vitamin C mg.
Apricots	217	4.3	54.6	72	98	2.1	4	1,198	11,510	0.14	0.16	2.6	42
Blackberries	250	5.2	55.6	138	82	3.9	4	733	860	0.14	1.18	1.6	90
Blueberries	259	2.9	63.8	63	54	4.2	4	338	420	0.13	0.25	1.9	58
Cherries, sour	242	5	59.7	92	79	1.7	8	797	4,170	0.21	0.25	1.7	42
Cranberries	200	1.7	47	61	44	2.2	9	357	190	0.13	0.09	0.4	47
Figs, fresh	363	5.4	92	159	100	2.7	9	880	360	0.29	0.24	1.9	7
Grapefruit	91	1.1	24	36	36	0.9	2	300	180	0.08	0.04	0.4	84
Grapes, white	270	2.4	69.8	48	81	1.6	12	698	400	0.21	0.11	1	18
Honeydew	94	2.3	22	40	46	1.1	34	717	120	0.13	0.09	1.8	65
Limes	107	2.7	36.2	126	69	2.3	8	389	50	0.10	0.08	0.7	141
Loquats	168	1.4	43.3	70	126	1.4	–	1,216	2,340	–	–	–	–
Oranges	162	3.3	40.4	136	66	1.3	3	662	660	0.33	0.13	1.3	166
Peaches	150	2.4	38.3	36	75	2	4	797	5,250	0.07	0.19	3.8	29
Pears	252	2.9	63.2	33	45	1.2	8	537	70	0.09	0.17	0.6	18
Pineapple	123	0.9	32.3	40	19	1.2	2	344	170	0.21	0.06	0.6	40
Plums	272	2.1	73.5	74	70	2.1	8	1,234	1,240	0.33	0.13	2.2	–
Prunes	1,018	8.4	269.1	204	315	15.6	32	2,770	6,390	0.35	0.66	6.3	12
Raspberries	321	6.6	69.1	132	97	4	4	876	trace	0.13	0.40	4	81
Strawberries	161	3	36.6	91	91	4.4	4	714	260	0.12	0.29	2.6	257
Tangerines	154	2.7	38.9	134	60	1.3	7	432	1,410	0.20	0.05	0.4	105
Watermelon	54	1	13.4	15	21	1	2	209	1,230	0.06	0.06	0.3	15

Figure 5-1

"RFF" ESTABLISHES REGULARITY DURING FASTING

The natural fruit acids stimulate the function of peristalsis (wave-like response, stimulated by the alternate contraction and relaxation of smooth muscle tissues of the gastro-intestinal tract) and help you establish regularity. This is essential since your metabolism is creating a form of internal combustion cell-slimming. Wastes need to be eliminated through the normal channels. When a raw fruit fast establishes regularity, these wastes are eliminated as part of your Slimfasting program. Many folks complain that reducing diets leave them constipated and, often, still overweight. On an RFF Slimfasting program, there is necessary regularity and, more important, swift weight loss.

"RFF" CREATES EXFOLIATE REACTION
FOR SWIFT SLIMMING

Fresh raw fruit introduced to your body's digestive system *without interference of other foods* can create an unusual *exfoliate reaction* that actually *dissolves the fat* right out of your adipose tissues. Sweet fruits are prime sources of enzymes that attack the fat in the cells and create this *exfoliate reaction* that strips away accumulated weight-causing wastes and helps create swift slimming.

"RFF" HAS UNIQUE SLIMFASTING POWER

Fresh raw fruits have this Slimfasting power because, botanically speaking, these foods are the edible portions of plants that result from the development of *pollinated flowers.* This process of pollination creates seed-bearing fruits which are prime sources of *levulose* (complete nature-created pre-digested sugar) which is ready for instant absorption and assimilation. This levulose triggers off a chain reaction within the metabolic block that enables the internal combustion process to literally burn up calories, carbohydrates and fats and slim down your body in a short time.

A raw fruit fast offers you appetite satisfaction, good health, as well as swift weight loss. It is considered an all-natural reducing pill.

How to Lose up to 45 Pounds
on an "RFF" Slimfasting Program

Joan W. needed desperately to lose up to 45 pounds. Not only did she show embarrassing bulges and unsightly inches, but she began to feel dizzy after the slightest exertion. Her breathing was labored. She feared developing diabetes (it ran in her family, she maintained) and heart trouble which had claimed the lives of her fat parents. But Joan W. found that while other diets did remove many unsightly pounds, she was left very weakened; also, she was troubled with constipation. Other diets also gave her a blotched skin, susceptibility to colds, and frequent headaches. She felt she could not cope with these side effects during an extended weight reducing program.

"RFF" KEEPS JOAN W.
"FIT AS A FIDDLE" AND "TWICE AS CURVY"

When she approached the RFF Slimfasting program, it was with many doubts and justified fears. She felt that it would leave her weak and more sensitive to other ailments. She complained that previous diets had caused the loss of many pounds but gave her these symptoms. But since she was desperate, she tried an eight day Raw Fruit Fast program. During these eight days, she ate nothing but a wide assortment of seasonal, fresh raw fruits. Results? She shed some 25 pounds. But more important, the RFF had no side effects for her. She boasted that she was "fit as a fiddle" throughout the fast and "twice as curvy" as she saw bulges and inches and pounds actually wash right out of her body. Afterwards, she resumed her usual eating but in modest portions. She skipped a week, then returned to another eight days of RFF Slimfasting and this time she said goodbye to the rest of the unwanted, unsightly 45 pounds.

YOUTHFUL, HEALTHY, ALERT

Joan W. not only slimmed down to a size 12, but she emerged from the RFF feeling youthful, with a healthy skin, bright, shining eyes, freedom from her allergies, and a clear head that was free of aches. She no longer felt dizzy and her breathing was refreshingly healthy. She had a neat "fiddle" figure that made her look and feel youthfully alert. The pounds not only were washed out of her body but they remained gone forever, thanks to the RFF program.

SCIENTISTS OFFER PROOF POSITIVE THAT FASTING WORKS

Joan W. approached reducing with some doubts. She researched the problem of overweight in the library. That was when she discovered there were hundreds of published scientific reports on fasting and how it could take off stubborn and "impossible" pounds when other programs were not too palatable. Joan W. was amazed to learn that thousands of people lost weight through fasting. Doctors and weight-loss specialists gave lectures and talks throughout the country on the benefits of fasting. It was frequently discussed on radio and television. Newspapers and magazines also carried stories on the effectiveness of fasting. So it was this increasing public awareness that made Joan W. go on a selected Slimfasting program. She joined the ranks of the tens of thousands who finally lost unwanted pounds by this popular method. Many came to fasting through the recommendation of friends, doctors, or reducing specialists.

Sample Raw Fruit Fast Program
for Swift Weight Loss

1. Plan ahead. Decide how many days of the RFF you wish to follow. Set a schedule.

2. Two days *before* your first day, eat only fruits or vegetables (cooked or raw) as your meals.

3. First day of your RFF eat a variety of different freshly washed, raw fresh fruits. Select any *seasonal* fruits. *Benefit:* If fruits are seasonal and permitted to ripen naturally, the sun and the life force of the tree or vine or bough combine to convert fruit starch into sugar. All this is done during the ripening process. When you eat the fully ripened fruit, you introduce natural fruit sugar (*levulose*) into your system. It requires *little or no digestion* on your part. This spares your metabolic system the labor which can then be used for utilizing the levulose and transporting nutrients and enzymes via the blood circulation to create the fat-splitting, cell-slimming reaction. *Suggestion:* Wherever possible, use fully ripened fruit for easy assimilation and digestive-sparing metabolism.

4. Second and subsequent days of your RFF should feature the same available variety of fresh raw fruits. Plan to eat three fruit meals daily. Your taste buds will not tire because each fruit has its own luscious good taste so variety will be your reward during an RFF Slimfasting program.

5. To break your fast, slowly ease into solid food. The first day after you have ended your RFF, you should have some steamed vegetables together with skim milk. The second day after you have ended your RFF should feature raw and steamed vegetables, skim milk products such as cottage cheese, and natural cheeses. The third day after your RFF, you may introduce a small portion of lean chicken or turkey as you gradually ease into your customary foods.

6. When you resume your usual eating patterns, you should have a reduced craving so that you can enjoy eating but *you will not overeat.* During the RFF Slimfasting program, the

intake of *levulose* helped put a natural control on your appetite and you now feel satisfied with less food.

7. Whenever possible, go on an RFF Slimfasting program so you can not only take off unwanted pounds but keep them off!

DIGESTIVE FREEDOM = SWIFT WEIGHT LOSS

The secret power of an RFF or raw fruit fast lies in its digestion-sparing power. Basically, weight loss calls for metabolic action upon the fat in your adipose cell tissues. But many heavy foods call for so much digestion that all efforts are directed toward that end. *Digestion cannot be used for attacking the fat in your adipose cell tissues since it is so fully occupied with attacking eaten food.*

But during a raw fruit fast, your digestion is spared efforts since nature has pre-digested the fruits which can be chewed, swallowed, enjoyed and assimilated with almost *no* digestive responsibility.

This liberates your digestion which can now turn to the process of elimination. That is, the attacking of the accumulated fats and other weight-causing globules that have fattened your adipose cell tissues. Then, the liberated digestive system is able to *eliminate* these weighty substances from your body. This helps create swift weight loss under a satisfying raw fruit fast.

"RFF" REJUVENATES, HEALS, CLEANSES

A raw fruit fast enables every organ of your body to switch into low gear, to help cast out unwanted weight. Furthermore, the RFF cleanses your billions of body cells, removing accumulated poisons and toxins (causes of ill health and overweight) and casting them out through your normal eliminative channels. This creates internal cleansing and purification that is rejuvenating.

A simple raw fruit fast will also help your body regroup and rebalance its resources and energies. In effect, this creates an *internal rebirth*. It is the all-purpose and all-inclusive way to remake yourself from head to toe, inside and outside, into a slim and youthfully healthy new person!

From "Hey, Fatty" to "Hi, Slim" in Ten Days

Andrew N. had endured taunts for more years than he cared to remember. He was not only overweight (the scales showed he weighed an excess 39 pounds) but he had unsightly jowls and a paunch that forced him to walk with the stooped gait of a man much older than his middle 40's. He had given up on many slimming programs because they left him tired, bored, hungry, weak. This last-named side effect of dieting made him discouraged in his battle to lose weight. He was an active salesman who had to be on the go all the time. He needed as much energy as possible, but dieting left him weak. So he felt resigned to being called "Hey, Fatty" instead of his dreamed-of, "Hi, Slim."

USES RAW FRUIT FAST FOR 10-DAY WEIGHT LOSS

Hearing of Slimfasting and how the digestive system can be turned into a self-programmed cell-slimming engine, Andrew N. decided to try a simple RFF program. He was told that the natural *levulose* in fruits would sweeten his blood sugar and give him the vital energy he needed while he shed those pounds that made him the object of scorn.

VITALITY, GLOWING HEALTH, SLIMMING DOWN

Andrew N. prepared for his RFF Slimfasting program by eating vegetables, either raw or cooked, two days before the fast. One day before the fast, he ate fruits, either raw or cooked. Then he began his RFF program and followed this method: *Breakfast:* Any assortment of different citrus fruits such as oranges, grapefruit wedges, seasonal berries. *Luncheon:* Any assortment of sweet fruits such as the banana, cherry, pear, plum, peach, melon, apple. *Dinner:* Mild fruits such as the pineapple, nectarine, date, grape, cantaloupe. *Nightcap:* Seasonal berries in their natural juices.

Within two days, Andrew N. noted that he was losing weight. Not only did his scale show the pounds being washed out of his body, but his belt was tightening. But more importantly, Andrew N. experienced youthful vitality and glowing health while on this raw fruit fast. He was on his toes, mentally and physically alert, with much vim and vigor as he continued his salesman's job throughout his 10-day Slimfasting program.

SLIM BODY, LOWERED WEIGHT, LEAN WAIST

By the end of his scheduled 10-day raw fruit fast program, his face and body had slimmed down so that he looked much younger than his so-called middle years. With the jowls and paunch gone, he walked erect. His waistline measured a youthful 30 inches! He was brimming with vitality and energy. The "RFF" program had *added* alertness and power to his body and mind. Now he was greeted as "Hi, Slim" as a reward for his easy efforts.

How to Buy Your Raw,
Fresh Fruits for Slimfasting

Note these guidelines:

Avoid Unripe Fruit. These contain carbohydrate substances and other forms of starch which require strong digestion and will place a burden on your own digestive system which distracts from essential cell-slimming. Unripe fruit is also unwholesome and unpalatable.

Avoid Overripe Fruit. These show signs of decay which can be toxic to your system; since the purpose of Slimfasting is to wash out toxic wastes, it is wise to avoid over-ripe fruits which can add toxic wastes. Furthermore, in an over-ripe fruit, the *levulose* has been changed into carbon dioxide, acetic acid and alcohol which makes it inharmonious to your health. There is much water loss that will dehydrate your system. Overripe fruit should be avoided.

Select Ripe Fruit. These are most luscious with good quality and flavor. They are healthfully alkaline with a proper amount of *levulose* as well as other vitamins, minerals, protein and enzymes that nourish your body and promote the action of *digestive-combustion* which will penetrate the thick coated membrane of your adipose cell tissues and help dissolve the fat to be washed out of your body to help you enjoy swift weight loss.

How to Use Your Raw,
Fresh Fruits for Slimfasting

Wash Thoroughly. Fresh fruits should always be washed before use, especially if they are not from an organic source. Wash under free running cold faucet water. Special fruit brushes (sold in houseware stores) may be used to further cleanse away any spray or other residue.

Chew Thoroughly. All fruit should be chewed very thoroughly. The act of chewing stimulates the flow of digestive enzymes that are needed to penetrate the strong membrane of the adipose cell tissues to get to the stored fat. So chew all fruits thoroughly. A good rule is to systematically liquefy every particle. This assures absorption and assimilation.

Room Temperature. Fruits should be eaten at ordinary room temperature. Avoid shocking your digestive system by gulping down refrigerated or ice-temperature fruit. This causes a sudden constriction of your digestive muscles and hinders absorption. Fruit should be of comfortable temperature as you chew and swallow.

Swallow Comfortably. Your chewed fruit should be swallowed comfortably. DO NOT gulp down huge chunks. Again, this forces your digestive system to tighten up and "fight" to accommodate the unnaturally large chunks. It is contrary to good assimilation. It will negate or refute all the hopes for internal combustion and cell-slimming.

FRESH RAW FRUITS THAT
HELP YOU SLIM DOWN SWIFTLY

When selecting fruits, try to obtain those that are in season. These have not undergone long storage or shipping time which may deplete their values. Select fresh *raw* fruits. While frozen, canned or bottled fruits may be used in certain unavoidable circumstances, they are not as effective as the fresh, raw variety. Here are some delicious fresh fruits that you can enjoy during your Slimfasting programs:

APPLES. Contain nutrients that will cleanse the vital organs. When taken on an empty stomach, the small amount of malic acid helps metabolize stubborn accumulations.

APRICOTS. Select tree-ripened apricots. Prime source of Vitamin A which is used by your metabolism to rebuild cells and tissues. Good iron source that helps enrich your bloodstream and keep you warm while pounds are melting away.

BANANAS. A prime source of important potassium which helps maintain a good blood and plasma condition as pounds are washed out of your system. Also helps to regulate the large intestine and maintain healthy bowel movements.

BERRIES. Very high in *levulose* which is used by your bloodstream to give you energy. The citric and malic acid in berries will act as cleansers for the tough membranes of the fat-containing cell. Can also act as starch-splitters to break up accumulated carbohydrates and thereby create weight loss.

CHERRIES. Good source of natural levulose as well as magnesium and silicon. These minerals are taken by your metabolism to keep your skin and skeletal structure in good health as weight is taken out of your body.

CRANBERRIES. High in sulphur as well as natural tannic acids, these nutrients are used by your metabolism to stimulate your pancreas so that sugar-metabolizing insulin is available to dissolve pounds.

CURRANTS. High in potassium which is used by your digestive system to help promote glandular hormones; also help cleanse the intestinal tract of mucous conditions. This internal scrubbing helps boost the power of self-combustion whereby the cells can be cleansed of fatty deposits.

DATES: A sweet fruit of the palm, it is higher in protein than most fruits and has a high mineral content. A very prime source of *levulose,* dates will energize your various systems and promote a feeling of alertness, vim and vigor. At the same time, date *levulose* will trigger your metabolic chain reaction to promote swifter *autolysis* (self-digesting) of cellular fats.

FIGS: Either white or dark, they are high in natural blood-building minerals. Help stimulate sluggish responses so that regularity is assured. Wastes and weighty toxic residues are thus propelled out of the body through the action of nutrients in figs.

GRAPES: Rich in blood-building iron and energizing *levulose,* grapes are strong in stimulating the processes whereby the fatty deposits are cleansed. They work to eliminate uric acid from the body, then help maintain an important acid-alkaline balance. This balance helps control the buildup of weight in the cells.

GRAPEFRUITS. High source of Vitamin C which is used by your metabolism to help dissolve accumulated deposits in the cartilage and joints. Bioflavonoids in the grapefruit are used to exhilarate the digestive system and digest "tough" and "stubborn" internal deposits.

LEMONS. A prime source of citric acid which is used by the metabolic system to break down accumulations during a Slimfasting program and wash them out of the system. Maintains a natural acid-alkaline balance which is a key to remaining slim.

MELONS (all varieties). Good source of potassium which is used to maintain cell fluid balance, permit nerve impulse conduction, and establish electrical potential. This penetrates the cells and helps wash out accumulated fatty deposits. *Suggestion:* Because melons are so all-purpose, it is often suggested that you go on a melon fast for good weight loss.

NECTARINES: A distinctive flavor reveals its high mineral content. It has a good balance of sodium and potassium which appears to stimulate the pancreas for more healthful sugar metabolism and natural slimming down.

OLIVES. Contain a natural fat that appears to penetrate stubborn deposits and "bathe" the adipose cells slimmingly clean. Very high in minerals that are needed to maintain a healthy bloodstream and to wash cells and keep them rejuvenated.

ORANGES. A prime source of natural fruit and citric acids, with essential vitamins and minerals. They create what is known as a "saprophytic reaction" which literally "explodes" stubborn fat and helps expel wastes and weight-causing elements. With an orange fast this saprophytic reaction can help keep you slim.

PAPAYAS. Known as "tree melons," they are prime sources of enzymes and digestive substances which can penetrate some of the strongest deposits of fats. Papyas grow on a giant herbaceous plant and when naturally ripened will offer a treasure of important minerals needed for blood health and for cellular rejuvenation.

PEACHES. Easily digested, the supply of natural hydrocyanic acid and fruit ethers give it an unusual vigorous strength to penetrate the membranes of fatty cells and loosen up wastes. During a Slim-fasting program, these substances of the peach are able to break down clumps and promote natural weight loss.

PEARS. A prime source of alkaline elements which act as a strong and *natural* diuretic so that accumulated sludge can be washed out of the system. High in *levulose*, pears energize the metabolic system to promote swifter weight loss.

PERSIMMONS. When fully ripened, they offer magnesium, phosphorus and potassium which are used to maintain cell fluid balance, establish electrical potential, permit nerve impulse conduction, utilize amino acids and set off an internal combustion that gives you good energy while the fat is being melted out of your body.

PINEAPPLES. A natural diuretic, the pineapple contains the bromelin enzyme which helps dissolve stubborn accumulations and then wash them out of your system.

PLUMS. Contain ingredients that establish regularity which is important in weight loss. Natural fruit sugars energize the metabolic system for swifter action during Slimfasting.

PRUNES. Considered a sweet fruit because it is about 70% levulose. It is this natural sugar that helps alert the digestive-eliminative systems to promote better internal combustion and waste removal.

RAISINS. Dried grapes, they are concentrated sources of vitamins, minerals and levulose which energizes the system so that both internally and externally you feel cleansed, alert, active.

TANGERINES. A citrus fruit, it is a good source of vitamins and minerals that act as corrosive agents to "burn away" strong deposits and help cleanse and reduce adipose fatty cells.

A raw fruit fast or RFF will set off a biological chain reaction within your system. It helps give you youthful energy while it creates spontaneous internal combustion that slims down the fat from your adipose storage cells.

Raw fruit also offers taste satisfaction, luscious eating pleasure and a feeling of comfort while you actually eat your way to a new slim figure.

SUMMARY

1. A raw fruit fast of a few days duration can help you lose unwanted and unnecessary pounds and inches from all parts of your body.

2. Raw fruit is an all-natural reducing pill. It will satisfy your chewing urge, nourish you, establish regularity, create exfoliate reaction and offer you unique Slimfasting.

3. Joan W. lost up to 45 pounds on an RFF Slimfasting program. She improved her health at the same time.

4. For swift weight loss, follow the easy Slimfasting program.

5. Andrew N. went from "Hey, Fatty" to "Hi, Slim" in 10 days with a raw fruit fast that made him energetic, vital and youthful while pounds and pounds and inches and inches just vanished from his body.

6. Follow the guidelines when buying and using raw fresh fruits for Slimfasting.

7. Enjoy Slimfasting with any of the variety of fruits available as listed in the mini-directory. Use singly or in combination for never-ending taste thrills and slimming results.

Chapter Six

Break the Pound Barrier
with a Raw Vegetable Fasting
("RVF") Program

Fresh raw vegetables are a prime source of nutrients that can help break through the stubborn pound barrier and create dramatic and swift weight loss. (See Figure 6-1.) Crisp vegetables offer chewing satisfaction as well as a feeling of fullness that eases and eliminates the problem of gnawing hunger pangs that interfere with many reducing programs.

SLIMFASTING WITH RAW VEGETABLES

To break the pound barrier, plan for a special and tasty RVF program whereby you devote one or more days per week to the intake of these succulent, raw, juicy plant foods. When you go on this delicious RVF or raw vegetable fasting program, here is how unique ingredients in these plant foods pierce through the pound barrier to create swift weight loss:

VITAMINS + ENZYMES = SELF-DIGESTION

Vitamins plus enzymes from vegetables work to create a self-digestion of accumulated fatty crystals within the intestinal tract; this relieves the efforts of the digestive glands which are now free to spark the process of "burning" known as *oxidation*. This is possible only through *raw* vegetables since cooking destroys the delicate vitamins and enzymes. Raw vegetables send a rich supply of these nutrients that are then activated through oxygen fixation to establish aerobic (forceful stream of oxygen) conditions in the intestinal-digestive tracts. This stimulates the formation of *coli bacteria* and causes their multiplication. The flourishing *coli bacteria* then have the power to metabolize, digest and eventually cause elimination of fat and weight

87

EDIBLE PORTION OF NUTRIENTS IN ONE POUND OF VEGETABLES

Vegetable	Calories	Protein grams	Carbohy-drate grams	Calcium mg.	Phos-phorus mg.	Iron mg.	Sodium mg.	Potas-sium mg.	Vitamin A I.U.	Thiamine mg.	Riboflavin mg.	Niacin mg.	Vitamin C mg.
Beets, no tops	137	5.1	31.4	51	105	2.2	190	1,064	80	0.10	0.15	1.2	32
Beet greens	61	5.6	11.7	302	102	8.4	330	1,448	15,490	0.24	0.55	1	76
Broccoli	113	12.7	20.9	364	276	3.9	53	1,352	8,840	0.35	0.81	3.2	400
Cabbage	98	5.3	22	200	118	1.6	82	530	530	0.22	0.20	1.3	192
Carrots	156	4.1	36.1	138	134	2.6	175	1,269	29,440	0.16	0.14	1.6	21
Cauliflower	122	12.2	23.6	113	254	5	59	1,338	270	0.50	0.44	3	354
Celery	58	3.1	13.3	133	95	1	429	1,160	820	0.09	0.11	1.2	30
Chard	104	10	19.2	367	163	13.4	613	2,295	27,120	0.25	0.72	2.2	132
Corn, raw	240	8.7	55.1	7	277	1.7	699	1,000	1,000	0.37	0.29	4.2	31
Cucumbers	46	2	10.6	56	60	1	20	530	0	0.11	0.14	0.7	37
Kale	154	17.4	26.1	723	270	7.8	218	1,097	29,030	0.47	0.76	6	540
Lettuce	47	4	8.4	117	87	6.7	30	886	3,200	0.21	0.20	0.9	28
Parsley	200	16.3	38.6	921	286	28.1	204	3,298	38,560	0.54	1.19	5.6	780
Peppers	82	4.5	17.9	33	82	2.6	48	792	1,540	0.28	0.30	2	476
Potatoes	279	7.7	62.8	26	195	2.2	11	1,495	trace	0.39	0.14	5.4	73
Radishes	69	4.1	14.7	122	127	4.1	73	1,314	40	0.13	0.12	1.3	106
Rhubarb (do not eat leaves)	62	2.3	14.4	374	70	3.1	8	979	390	0.12	0.26	1.2	34
Spinach	118	14.5	19.5	422	231	14.1	322	2,132	36,740	0.44	0.91	2.8	231
Squash (summer)	84	4.8	18.5	123	128	1.8	4	889	1,800	0.23	0.38	4.5	95
Tomatoes	100	5	21.3	59	122	2.3	14	1,107	4,080	0.29	0.18	3	102
Turnips	117	3.9	25.7	152	117	2	191	1,045	trace	0.16	0.26	2.2	140
Turnip greens	127	13.6	22.7	1,116	263	8.2	—	high	34,470	0.94	1.78	3.4	628
Watercress	79	9.2	12.5	630	225	7.1	217	1,177	20,450	0.35	0.68	3.6	330

Figure 6.1

throughout the body. *This is possible only when raw vegetables, containing vitamins and enzymes, are made available.* These nutrients are able to establish this aerobic condition which, literally, dissolves the fat out of the body. A tasty "RVF" program can help create this system.

GREEN LEAFY FOODS SUCH AS VEGETABLES CREATE FAT MOBILIZING ACTION

Within the "veins" of green leaves and most raw vegetables are vitamins, minerals, protein that create what is regarded as a fat mobilizing action. One pound of vegetables (see chart in this chapter) will give you many of those needed nutrients that can help metabolize, dissolve and then wash fatty substances out of your body. These nutrients promote the formation of red blood cells, stimulate respiration and nitrogen metabolism of your adipose cell tissues, alert your pancreas to issue more sugar-dissolving insulin, improve general circulation. These methods are able to attack the fat in your adipose cell tissues and create quick weight loss.

INTERNAL COMBUSTION ACTION FOR WEIGHT REDUCTION

The nutrients in raw vegetables restore a favorable acid-alkaline balance of the ashes after food combustion. This creates quick weight loss. It is more effective if your digestive system is NOT burdened by the presence of cooked foods and other foods that would detract from the task of assimilating these vegetables. When raw vegetables on a simple RVF Slimfasting program become the total intake, then the process of internal combustion can work fully to create the fat melting response for swift weight loss.

How to Lose up to 39 Pounds and Six Inches on an RVF Program

Peter F. was given a choice: Lose up to 39 pounds and six inches or face the risk of a serious illness. But Peter F. had gone the route of many other diets. They did work. They did lose many of his pounds. But he was always hungry, always had growling stomach pains, complained of feeling weak. No sooner did he go off his diet, than he would start eating to make up for "lost time" and the pounds would accumulate, the inches would start expanding. So Peter F. faced a difficult choice. He could lose weight and avoid possible illness; but when he finished his diet, he knew he would regain the lost and unwanted pounds and inches. It was a vicious dieting circle. He felt hopeless.

"RVF" PROGRAM IS TASTY, HEALTHFUL, SLIMMING

A Slimfasting program consisting of raw vegetables appealed to Peter F. He felt it would be satisfying and he decided to try it. His simple program:

Every Monday, Wednesday and Friday he would devote exclusively to the eating of seasonal, fresh raw vegetables. He would eat as much as he wanted of these raw vegetables for his three daily meals. For the rest of the week, he could eat whatever else he wanted.

Results? Within 14 days, he was able to lose about 25 pounds; his waistline began to slenderize; inch after inch was melted away from his waistline and other body parts. By the time he had finished his third week, Peter F. had lost the unwanted, undesirable 39 pounds; his waistline was trim, since the bulging six inches had also been taken off.

Peter F. was delighted not only with the swift weight loss, but with his feeling of satisfaction; he had no hunger or growling pains. When he lost his desired excess weight and pounds, he decided to keep them off by going on an RVF or raw vegetable fast every single Wednesday. He also discovered that his previously uncontrollable appetite was now under easy and effortless self-control. He felt satisfied with smaller food portions. He looked and felt youthfully healthy, thanks to this chewy good Slimfasting program.

Sample Raw Vegetable Fast Program
for Swift Weight Loss

1. Plan ahead. Schedule the number of days per week that you will use the RVF program. Mark it on your calendar.

2. Two days *before* your first RVF day, eat a variety of different fruits or vegetables (cooked or raw) for your meals.

3. First day of your RVF eat a variety of different freshly washed raw vegetables. Wherever possible, select seasonal vegetables. *Benefits:* Fully vine- or bough-ripened vegetables have vitamins, minerals and proteins of the highest quality. They are a prime source of natural enzymes which have the ability to melt the most stubborn fat deposits throughout the body. Seasonal and naturally ripened vegetables contain *volatile carbohydrates* which have the unique power of *catabolism.* It is this built-in power that uses carbohydrates to help digest and then dissolve accumulated fats. It is when vegetables are over-ripened or cooked that the carbohydrates become *sluggish*

and weak. They cannot create their fat-melting catabolism-action. They may cause weight gain. To avoid this, vegetables should be fresh, raw and, wherever possible, naturally ripened so the *volatile carbohydrates* (strong and powerful enzyme-containing vegetables) can use their *catabolism-action* for more effective and swift weight loss.

4. Second and subsequent days of your RVF should feature any available variety of seasonal, fresh raw vegetables. Plan to eat three such meals daily. You will discover a never-ending joy in raw vegetables because of so many varieties, colors, tastes.

5. To break your RVF program, slowly ease into solid foods. The first day after you have ended your RVF, begin with some steamed vegetables together with skim milk. Feature a raw or slightly cooked fruit dish for one meal during the day. The second day after you have ended your RVF, introduce some steamed brown rice, and also steamed vegetables. Also plan for one raw and/or cooked fruit meal. Add some skim milk products such as cottage cheese, natural cheeses. The third day after your RVF you may enjoy a small portion of lean turkey with some brown rice and a fresh fruit platter. You may also have chicken, if you prefer.

6. When you resume your usual eating patterns, you will notice a lowered craving for food. You will enjoy most of your favorite foods but with smaller though satisfying portions.

7. Whenever possible, go on an RVF Slimfasting program to give you chewy good satisfaction as the pounds and inches just roll off.

RAW VEGETABLE ENZYMES = QUICK "INCHES AWAY" WEIGHT LOSS

Raw vegetables contain enzymes, those protein-like substances that are so powerful, they are able to digest the toughest membranes. Enzymes are activators within the digestive system. They create a form of metabolism so that the tough membrane and the stubborn fat that acts as a barrier can be pierced, broken through, dissolved and then eliminated from the system.

To create this breaking of the pound barriers, your body needs raw, uncooked vegetables that can be taken up by your digestive system and metabolized so that enzymes are removed for use in fat-melting.

During a Raw Vegetable Fast, your digestive system is spared the competition or interference from other foods. Therefore, it is free and liberated. It can devote *full attention* to the use of enzymes to pound away at the fat deposits in your adipose cell tissues, to break them down and remove them. Under this process, the raw vegetable enzymes can create quick "inches away" weight loss while you eat to your satisfaction of all available vegetables.

SELF-CLEANSING, REJUVENATING, SLIMMING

Enzymes also act as "brooms" whereby they scrub the billions of body cells and tissues, helping to alert your circulation to wash these cells and permit *collagen,* a natural cement-like substance, to be used to repair and renovate them. This creates a feeling of rejuvenation. There is a simultaneous slimming down as the waste products, such as accumulated fats, are actually washed right out of your system. A periodic RVF is the natural way to rejuvenate and slim down.

From a Matron to a Mademoiselle in Ten Days

Maude O. bemoaned the fact that her mirror told her she looked like a middle-aged matron. She had heavy facial features, thick upper arms, a sagging throatline. Her heavy bust and hips made her walk with a stooped gait so that she looked (and felt) like an oldish matronly woman. Maude O. knew that it was her urge to snack and nibble all the time that had put on more than 35 pounds, not to mention the unsightly bulges that made her look unpleasingly plump and middle-aged. If she could only find a reducing program that would make her feel filled up even as she slimmed down, she would be happy. A nutritionist friend advised fasting, and Maude turned to the raw vegetable fast program because it would enable her to nibble while she lost weight.

NIBBLES, MUNCHES, SLIMS DOWN

Maude O. followed a simple but most effective program. She would eat her favorite foods during most of the week. But *the middle days of the week* were devoted to her RVF program wherein she would eat only vegetables—but *all* the vegetables she wanted.

She could nibble celery chunks, sliced radishes, turnip wedges, carrot slices, even raw lettuce and cabbage slices. For flavor, she would dip them into a bit of skim milk cottage cheese and sprinkle them with onion or garlic powder. This satisfied her insatiable nibbling and munching urge but did NOT add pounds.

Benefits: Chewing the vegetables triggered off her digestive enzyme system whereby important substances concentrated solely upon the added fat that had deposited itself all over her body. The very act of chewing is important in some situations of stubborn fat. Chewing increases the flow of gastric juices that are needed to metabolize accumulated fat. The gastric juices took up the vitamins and minerals of the raw vegetables and used them to break down the pound barriers by initiating action to dissolve pounds and thereby cause a loosening and elimination of these weighty wastes.

Loses 24 Pounds, 7 Inches. Before 10 days were over, Maude O. had delightfully lost some 24 pounds. Her tape measure showed that 7 inches had gone from her middle. When she looked into the mirror, her face was slenderized, her arms were lean, her throatline was firm. Now that the heavy and weighty pounds and inches had gone from her bust and hips so that she could walk erect, her carriage was like that of a young person. She delighted in the easy RVF wherein she would Slimfast on raw vegetables every Tuesday, Wednesday, Thursday and eat normally the rest of the week. It curtailed her nibbling urge. It helped her enjoy most of her favorite foods but in smaller portions. Within ten days, Maude O. had gone from a matron to a slim mademoiselle!

How to Buy Your Raw, Fresh Vegetables for Slimfasting

Note these guidelines:

Avoid Unripe Vegetables. These are not yet fully mature and their supply of vitamins, minerals, proteins and enzymes are weak. They will not provide sufficient vigor for internal combustion for fast fat-melting action.

Avoid Overripe Vegetables. The natural carbohydrate content has been overripened and there is more sugar present than any other nutrient. These vegetables are often weak since the enzyme content has been used up during the process of ripening the vegetable until it has little value left for slimming you down.

Select Ripe Vegetables. In particular, these are good ripe vegetables and have excellent Slimfasting benefits:

Leaves—spinach, chard, beet greens, turnip greens, cabbage, mustard greens, kale, cabbage, all lettuce. *Benefits:* The "veins" of these leaves are prime sources of enzymes and nutrients that can help liquefy accumulated fats while nourishing you at the same time.

Roots and Tubers—potatoes, sweet potatoes, turnips, radishes,

salsify, parsnips, onions. *Benefits:* Prime source of natural carbohydrates which have a corrosive action on the stubborn pound
barriers and can help break down the accumulations.

Buds and Flowers—broccoli, cauliflower, Brussels sprouts.
Benefits: The need for chewing stimulates gastric juices which work
freely during a fast (without other interfering foods) to help slim
down the fat cells. Chewing also offers good mouth satisfaction and
soothes the nibbling urge.

Seeds—beans, peas, peanuts, okra, lima, lentils. (Some steaming
is required to make beans and peas palatable.) *Benefits:* These plant
foods release nutrients that have "magnetic" action and attract
wastes and debris, carry them to eliminative channels and cast them
out of the body. Metabolism then uses these plant foods to provide
needed bulk and elimination during Slimfasting.

Fruits—tomatoes, green peppers, cucmbers, squash, eggplant,
pumpkin. Called "fruits" since they are the "blossoms" of the
vegetable plant. *Benefits:* Prime sources of vitamins, minerals, proteins and "blossomed" nutrients which are at the peak of their
power. Help to penetrate thick membranes during a Slimfasting
program for dissolution and eventual elimination.

How to Use Your Fresh, Raw Vegetables for Slimfasting

Wash Thoroughly. Raw vegetables should always be washed under free running cold water especially if not from an organic source.
Special vegetable brushes (sold in houseware stores) may be used to
further cleanse away any spray residues.

Steam Slightly. Some raw vegetables such as potatoes, beans,
peas should be steamed slightly since you could not otherwise eat
them. Use a steamer basket (available in houseware stores and health
food shops) to gently steam the vegetables and make them chewy
good with no loss of nutrients.

Chew Thoroughly. Always chew your vegetables very
thoroughly. This alerts the flow of digestive juices. This also unlocks
and releases the stored up nutrients in the vegetable and makes them
readily available for nourishment and slimming down. *Suggestion:*
Chew leisurely and thoroughly until of a smooth blenderized quality
and then swallow.

Room Temperature. Avoid eating vegetables that are too cold or
too hot. Do not gulp. Let the vegetable remain at room temperature
a few moments and then partake. This will be soothing to your
system.

Swallow Comfortably. After you have thoroughly chewed your vegetable, swallow it comfortably. Avoid swallowing big chunks. Do not swallow quickly. If you do, your gastro-intestinal system reacts with a shock and there is an excessive outpouring of hydrochloric acid that may "rebound" up your esophagus (food gullet) and cause burning. This negates the digestive principle. This tends to upset your homeostasis (body balance) and Slimfasting is ineffective. So eat and swallow with comfort and joy for better health and more effective Slimfasting.

FRESH RAW VEGETABLES FOR SWIFT WEIGHT LOSS

Vegetables should, preferably, be consumed during the season. Try to avoid those that are out of season since they are depleted because of incomplete growth, long storage or shipping times. Wherever possible, these vegetables should be *raw.* You may want to use frozen, canned or bottled vegetables, if nothing else is available. But these have been pre-cooked and some nutrients have been evaporated away during the process. So the rule of thumb is to use raw vegetables wherever and whenever possible. Here are many delicious fresh raw vegetables to be enjoyed during your Slimfasting programs:

ALFALFA. During thorough chewing, there is a release of alkaline substances which soothe the gnawing hunger pains, provide a feeling of satisfaction while weight is slowly going down.

ASPARAGUS. Contains minerals that act as cleansers of the vital body organs, freeing them of accumulated wastes so slimming can occur through better function.

BEETS. Prime source of nutrients that will cleanse the liver, nourish the hemoglobin (red coloring matter of the bloodstream) and dissolve excessive wastes that might otherwise build up unwanted pounds.

BROCCOLI. High in minerals that help create a better acid-alkaline medium within the digestive system so that autolysis is more effective and weight is more easily lost.

CABBAGE. High Vitamin A content helps boost iron metabolism to enrich the bloodstream and keep you warm while pounds are shed.

CARROTS. High potassium and other mineral content, together with a carotene—a substance that transforms into Vitamin A. This reaction is helpful for cleansing the system and promoting weight loss. The Vitamin A also helps to boost calcium absorption.

CAULIFLOWER. Good source of protein which becomes transformed into amino acids that work to catalyse fat and slim down the adipose cell tissues and promote weigh loss; also offers a feeling of bulk while you slim down.

CELERY. The dark green leaves contain a "plant hormone" that is believed to activate the pancreas to secrete needed insulin so that sugar can be better "burned." It thereby creates swift weight loss while you chew your way to a new slim figure. Minerals in the celery also ease your appestat or "hunger clock" so you feel relaxed while you reduce! Fiber contained in celery creates needed bulk to maintain regularity.

CHIVES. Act as natural diuretic which is essential in helping liquefy your system so that melted down fatty accumulations can then be washed out.

CUCUMBERS. Good source of hair and skin building minerals so that you look youthful with good health while you slim down. While cucumber skin is a prime source of digestants, you should not eat it unless you are guaranteed that it is of an organic source.

ENDIVE. Helps "scrape" off the accumulations from your organs because of its high mineral and enzyme content. Use regularly.

FENNEL. Contains nutrients that are alkalizing; help to loosen "mucus" and "glue" which causes overweight. Acts as a natural diuretic to wash out these accumulations.

KALE. Eaten raw, a potent source of enzymes that will help boost metabolism and increase the excretion of weighty wastes.

LETTUCE. All varieties are good sources of nutrients that act as sparkplugs to the metabolic system. Helps wash the cells and tissues by providing potassium and water and loosen accumulations.

MUSTARD GREENS. High in sulphur and phosphorus which promote "washing" of the digestive-intestinal tracts and keep them clean so they can create necessary substances for good metabolism.

OKRA. Combine with other raw vegetables to help soothe the internal organs and promote regularity. Helps to increase powers of elimination for better slimming.

ONIONS. Contain naturally strong substances that help cleanse the mucous and cellular membranes for more effective slimming. Use chopped or sliced Spanish onions as part of a raw salad for a delectable taste and strong internal cleansing.

PARSLEY. Contains vitamins, minerals, protein that promote oxygen metabolism to help maintain better health of the liver, as well as adrenal and thyroid glands. It helps cleanse wastes and also helps eliminate excessive uric acid.

PARSNIPS. The water in parsnips will help cleanse the bladder, kidneys and other organs so that they can function more efficiently.

PEPPERS. High Vitamin A and C content make peppers important for body metabolism, which needs these nutrients for activation.

POTATOES. Steam potatoes slightly so you do not increase the starch content. If potatoes remain at room temperature for a few days before cooking, their natural carbohydrate content is increased. Then use as part of a raw salad to help improve metabolism, nourish the system.

PUMPKIN. Soothing to the various organs, it acts as a natural diuretic in washing out pound-causing wastes.

RADISHES. Appear to help dissolve accumulated mucus and "glue" due to high water content and then stimulate the entire digestive system so that cleansing is more effectively achieved. The skin contains substances which make the natural water an "antiseptic" for internal cleansing.

SQUASH. Prime source of Vitamin A, which can nourish the body while you slim down.

TOMATOES. High vitamin content will help nourish the freshly washed cells and tissues and help protect against unnecessary build-up of weight.

TURNIPS. The high content of Vitamin A and Calcium is good to help strengthen your skeletal structure while pounds are being washed away.

WATERCRESS. A strong intestinal cleanser because of high sulphur, phosphorus and chlorine content. It helps dissolve coagulated blood fibrin in hemorrhoids and protect as well as relieve such problems. A good source of body building minerals.

During an RVF Slimfasting program in which you control intake of food so that vegetables are consumed exclusively, you will be chewing a great deal. This insures proper salivation, flow of digestive enzymes, the automatic cleansing of your system through this action. You will also feel comfortable, full, satisfied, with minimal (if any) hunger pangs as you are able to be nourished while Slimfasting!

IMPORTANT HIGHLIGHTS

1. Break the stubborn pound barrier with a raw vegetable fast that offers vitamins + enzymes to create self-digestion of accumulated fats and weight-causing wastes.

2. Green leaves of raw vegetables contain substances that create a fat mobilizing action, as well as internal combustion for good weight reduction.

3. Peter F. lost up to 39 pounds and six inches on a simple RVF program that let him feel filled up while he slimmed down.

4. Follow the easy step-by-step program for a raw vegetable fast.

5. Maude O. went from a "matron" to a "mademoiselle" in ten days with an easy 3 days per week raw vegetable fast. Lost inches, pounds, bulges. Regained youth.

6. Buy good vegetables for good results. Follow instructions.

7. Note how to use and enjoy a garden of different raw vegetables for swift, effective and "no fault" weight loss.

Chapter Seven

The High Fiber Fast ("HFF") Way to Magic Weight Loss

A simple everyday food has the ability to make you feel filled up, comfortably satisfied while the pounds and inches melt away from your body. That food is *fiber*. Also known as *roughage* or *cellulose,* it is nature's own method for creating a "time release" reaction whereby you will feel hunger satisfaction along with a natural decline in appetite. This biological response will help put a self-control on your urge to eat and the pounds will actually slip right out of your body as the hours and days go on . . . *with no effort or strain on your part.*

What Is Fiber? It is a term for plant material that your body does not digest. It passes through your body after it is eaten and is then eliminated. Fiber is found in the cell walls of most plant foods. It is the portion of the plant cell wall that largely resists digestion. Fiber creates *bulk* within your system and this gives you a feeling of fullness so that you will naturally eat less and lose weight.

Where Is Fiber Found? In plant foods such as grains, vegetables fruits, nuts and seeds. Fiber is not found in animal foods. The most potent source of fiber is found in bran.

What Is Bran? It is the outermost layer of the grain seed or kernel. This part of the wheat kernel also contains a major share of important nutrients such as vitamins, minerals, protein.

What Are Good Sources of Bran? Unprocessed and unrefined natural wheat cereal products sold in many supermarkets and health stores. Pure bran, itself, is the best source of natural fiber. It is cholesterol-free and low in fat. This makes it advantageous on a cholesterol-fat controlled eating program.

What Are Some Non-Grain Sources of Fiber? Fresh raw fruits and vegetables as well as most seeds and nuts offer good amounts of fiber, but not as much as in non-processed wheat products as well as bran. Sun-dried fruits are also good sources of fiber but high in calories so should be eaten sparingly.

Known as "roughage" or "bulk," fiber is a simple food that has the amazing power of being able to create magic weight loss.

10 MAGIC WEIGHT LOSING POWERS
OF A HIGH FIBER FAST

When you use ordinary bran as your source of fiber (along with fruits and vegetables as well as seeds and nuts) on a simple but magically effective Slimfasting program, these 10 "magic weight losing powers" occur to take off pounds and inches, *almost overnight:*

1. Fiber creates a sponge-like bulk in the system that has the unique ability to absorb fluid. This will create a natural "appetite-control" that offers hunger-satisfaction and a lowered desire for higher calorie foods.

2. Fiber reduces the transit time of food passing through your intestinal tract. This tends to reduce the amount of calories your body receives from foods that you eat.

3. Fiber tends to stabilize your process of metabolism by restoring your balance to a part-fiber, part-nutrient composition. This tends to improve the metabolic powers of your digestive system so there is *better internal combustion for burning up of stored up and excessive calories and fats so you lose more unwanted pounds.*

4. Fiber foods are crisp, chewy and crunchy to eat. When you eat natural brown rice, a broth or soup containing much bran, crisp vegetables, fresh apples, you need time and energy to chew and absorb. This gives you good chewing satisfaction; this also helps use up much energy during the eating and swallowing and digestion process and more calories are burned up in the process. In effect, *eating fiber foods is like "exercising" your digestive system and burning up calories.*

5. Fiber foods offer much natural roughage or bulk. When you have eaten a bowl of crisp vegetables, lettuce and sliced radishes, you experience good appetite satisfaction and less of a desire to eat slushy foods.

6. Fiber foods require much chewing. This produces an increased flow of salivary and gastric enzymes which combine with food in the stomach and causes a swelling of food fibers. Automatically, the stomach becomes distended and there is that important feeling of *fullness* that makes reducing a comfortable joy.

7. Fiber foods appear to put a control on the ability of the small intestine to absorb and store calories. This means

that on a high fiber fast or HFF program, you can eat more, and pounds will be lost. *Note:* Caloric storage in the small intestine is a forerunner to excessive weight gain since this organ will then distribute these calories to other body parts. This causes unsightly bulges and inches.

8. Fiber helps to create more regularity. Many dieters complain of constipation during a slimming program. Not so when fiber-creating roughage is part of your program. Furthermore, a high fiber fast program helps you excrete more fat with each movement than if you were on a low fiber program. When you follow an HFF program, you are actually excreting a good portion of excess body fat as each day passes on.

9. Fiber lets you nibble and chew to offer "oral satisfaction" throughout the day while you do not risk gaining unwanted pounds.

10. Fiber feeds your digestive system important vitamins, minerals, proteins that are used to nourish your organs and give you good health and protection from intestinal ailments while you lose weight.

An HFF program lets you enjoy many of your favorite foods, even so-called forbidden sweets, if you have that craving, while you lose unwanted pounds and inches.

BASIC HIGH FIBER FAST PROGRAM FOR "OVERNIGHT" WEIGHT LOSS

Rose D. wanted to lose weight *fast*. She was anxious to shed the 39 excess pounds that stubbornly clung to her hips, thighs, as well as her upper arms and shoulders. No matter how hard she tried, Rose D. could not get rid of those unsightly pounds. Other reducing programs were helpful but they often made her constipated. Or else, they could not ease the gnawing hunger pangs that kept her awake all night until she had to "raid the refrigerator" and stuff herself so much that when she weighed herself the next day, the scales were higher than ever! So Rose D. turned to the high fiber fast program with hope for a symptom-free Slimfasting plan that would make her feel filled up while pounds melted away swiftly.

BRAN + EVERYDAY FOODS = WEIGHT LOSS

Rose D. supplied herself with bran which she purchased from her local health store. It was unrefined and non-processed. Then she stocked up on her favorite foods. Here is the simple "HFF" program that Rose D. followed that helped melt away more than 39 extra pounds and many inches, *almost overnight:*

BREAKFAST

Bran Tonic: 2 teaspoons of whole bran stirred into a full glass of grapefruit or orange juice.

Fresh Fruit: Fresh raw apple or pear or orange or a bowl of seasonal berries with a dollop of skim milk cottage cheese.

Cereal: One serving of shredded wheat or whole bran or granola in skim milk with a half teaspoon of honey.

Toast: Made of 100% whole wheat bread.

Beverage: Coffee substitute such as Postum or any herb tea with some skim milk and honey.

LUNCHEON

Bran Tonic: 2 teaspoons of whole bran stirred into a full glass of tomato juice.

Protein Food: Lean turkey or chicken or small slices of roast beef on 100% whole wheat bread.

Vegetables: Bowl of lettuce and tomato with sliced green peppers and carrot sticks.

Dessert: Melon wedges or fresh peach halves with a small drizzle of honey, if desired.

Beverage: Coffee substitute such as Postum or any herb tea with some skim milk and honey.

DINNER

Bran Tonic: 2 teaspoons of whole bran stirred into a full glass of carrot or celery juice or any desired vegetable juice.

Soup: Split green pea soup into which is stirred a half teaspoon of bran.

Protein Food: Broiled turkey or chicken. (Remove fat from beneath skin.)

Grain: Brown rice with onion or garlic powder flavoring.

Vegetable: Corn on the cob or steamed squash.

Dessert: Seasonal fresh berries (not canned or frozen since these are laden with sugar) with a small portion of skim milk and a drizzle of honey.

BEDTIME SNACK

Yogurt into which you have stirred some bran. *Slimfasting Benefit:* The yogurt adds *lactobacillus* bacteria, a substance which cleanses the intestinal tract. It also helps destroy potentially harmful bacteria in the tract through a detoxifying action. It also helps establish more alertness to the intestinal tract. This boosts the easy and speedy elimination of weight-causing fat from your body.

NO HUNGER PANGS, NO CONSTIPATION, NO STARVATION

Rose D. followed the preceding HFF Slimfasting program with delicious enjoyment. There were no hunger pangs, constipation or starvation. Almost immediately, she discovered her weight going down! The scales showed that pounds were literally being "cast out" of her body. Encouraged by this fully comfortable Slimfasting program, she continued for 24 days. At the end of her schedule, she discovered that she had lost *more* than her unwanted 39 pounds. She had shed some 47 pounds!

LOOKS, FEELS, ACTS YOUNGER

Added benefits were that the weighty "clumps" were washed away from her hips, thighs, upper arms and shoulders. Her chin line firmed up, too. Her face was smooth and firm. Her body contours were shapely. Everyone told Rose D. that she was rejuvenated! With the overweight gone, Rose D. looked, felt and acted much younger. She could even go square dancing with the vitality and joy of a youngster. She was now a slim-trim 112 pounds. Slimfasting had created that magic weight loss . . . forever!

THE FIVE-CENT FOOD
THAT IS WORTH A MILLION DOLLARS

Bran fiber costs less than 5¢ per day and yet is worth a million dollars because it creates the internal swelling and improved metabolism that leads to miracle weight loss. All this and much, much more for just 5¢ per day.

How Much Fiber Is Needed? It is believed that 7 grams daily will set off the metabolic chain reaction that is needed to create weight loss. You may want to take more than this minimum.

What Is Best Source of Fiber? Whole unprocessed bran is the richest source of fiber. It contains about 4.7 grams per each cup.

What Is a Good Plan for Fiber Intake? Take about 6 tablespoons of bran daily. Distribute these amongst your meals. Eat some fiber with each meal. This will give your digestive system a "time-release" supply so that metabolism will keep churning away to create better combustion and regular weight loss around the clock, even while you sleep!

Yes, this simple 5¢ food can give you a "million dollar" reducing miracle while you enjoy most of your favorite foods.

HOW TO USE BRAN IN DAILY MENU PLANNING

Here are some easy ways to get your daily supply of bran:

1. Sprinkle it over any dry whole grain breakfast cereal with skim milk and some fresh fruit.
2. Add bran to a whole grain cereal that requires cooking— before or after.
3. Get into the custom of stirring one tablespoon of bran with fruit juice.
4. Stir one tablespoon of bran into vegetable juice.
5. Mix it into skim milk yogurt, plain or flavored.
6. Add it to soups.
7. Combine with sauce or gravy.
8. Sprinkle it over salad, fruit or vegetable, and combine with any salad dressing.
9. When making stuffed peppers, meat loaf or casserole, add some bran.
10. When baking bread or whole grain pastries or cakes, add some bran.

HOW TO LOSE WEIGHT ON AN "HFF" MEAT AND POTATOES PROGRAM

Nicholas Z. was a "meat and potatoes" man who needed to slim down. But he refused to give up his huge portions of food, including his beloved meat and potatoes, not to mention other fattening foods. Only when he began to experience dizzy spells and heavy breathing because of corpulence, did he realize he would have to heed his family's urgings to lose weight. But he had tried conventional reducing diets with mixed results and, therefore, was skeptical that he could stick to a diet. He had previously lost weight but suffered because he had to give up his beloved "meat and potatoes" and customary heavy, fattening foods. He grudgingly consented to a high fiber fast program, if only to prove to his wife and family that it would not work and that maybe he could survive with his excessive appetite and excessive weight.

SLIMFASTING WITH HEAVY FOODS

His wife made a few changes, ever mindful that she wanted to satisfy Nicholas' eating urges while slimming him down. Here is the HFF program that saved Nicholas' life, satisfied his appetite, and caused some 49 overweight pounds to "vanish."

1. Meat was trimmed fat-free.

2. Mashed potatoes were prepared with a built-in reducing substance. This was done by first boiling two tablespoons of bran for about ten minutes. In another kettle, potatoes were boiled, until soft. Then, the excess water was drained from the bran mixture. The bran was then mashed or whipped together with the potatoes. *Benefit:* The fiber in the bran swelled up during digestion and *speeded up* transit time of the potatoes so that they arrived in the colon early, and then there was a short layover in the colon and prompt evacuation with *bile acids intact.* This reduced "layover" of the potatoes meant that the intestinal tract had a correspondingly reduced opportunity to take any calories and carbohydrates for storage and subsequent weight gain. The quicker the removal of starch-sugar-fat foods, the less storage of carbohydrates, calories and fats and less or even no weight gain!

3. In many meat dishes, Nicholas' wife also mixed bran so that there would be a high fiber intake; this fiber would then work to create swift transit time with reduced opportunity for removal of weight-causing elements. Therefore, the "meat and potatoes" lover could feast while fasting his way to a slim-trim shape.

EATS HEARTILY, LOSES POUNDS, INCHES

Nicholas Z. ate heartily, while he started to lose 5, 10, 15 and as much as 49 pounds. His waistline started to shrink. Soon, *ten inches* had been taken off. His once flabby thighs were now firm. He could breathe easily. His dizzy spells ended. More important, on this high fiber fast program, the pounds and inches not only went off, *they stayed off permanently.*

HOW TO SLIMFAST WITH WHOLE GRAIN BREAD

Since fiber is the key to speeded-up transit time of food in the system, it is possible to Slimfast with whole grain bread products.

When these grain foods enter your digestive system, the fiber content acts as a "starter engine" to alert the metabolic system to speed up assimilation and eventual elimination. Fiber, in whole grains, can help you slim down while you enjoy your favorite bread products. Here are some whole grain products that you can enjoy and slim down with:

BULGUR. Also known as parboiled wheat or wheat pilaf. It is made by "cracking" or breaking the whole wheat kernel or berry instead of grinding it. *How to Use:* As a cooked cereal, as a replacement for rice or potatoes, mixed with other grains for bread or cake baking.

BARLEY. A cereal grass. Select whole grain barley. Do *not* use "pearled" or "polished" barley since this means much of the valuable bran or fiber has been removed. *How to Use:* Add to casseroles, soups, stews, or cooked cereals.

BUCKWHEAT. Seeds of the buckwheat plant, hulled or made into groats or flour. Also in the form of kasha. This nut-flavored grain is also available as "buckwheat groats" which are the whole, hulled kernels. *How to Use:* Available as buckwheat flour for use in baking. Combine with other grains or use alone for breads, muffins, waffles, cookies, rolls, etc. Also use as a cereal.

MILLET. A seed grain with an alkaline ash which tends to balance the ash of acid secretions so that metabolism is improved and calories are burned much more quickly. *How to Use:* Combine millet with other grains. Serve by itself for a delicious cereal. Creamy yellow, millet seeds offer a firm and pleasant texture to casseroles.

RICE. Select *only* the whole, unpolished *brown* rice for good fiber content. In brown rice, only the outer, inedible fibrous husk has been removed. *How to Use:* Cooked brown rice is delicious as an accompaniment to any dish. Also use as stuffing or filling, in soups, casseroles.

CORN. Select non-degerminated corn flour. Avoid "instant" or "degerminated" since the nutrient-filled germ containing the fiber has been removed to extend shelf life. Use white or yellow non-degerminated corn meal or flour. This has been made by grinding corn kernels to medium meal consistency on buhrstones (a siliceous rock used for millstones). *How to Use:* As a flour for making breads, rolls, muffins, hotcakes, tamale pies, fritters, scrapple.

OATS. Select the natural hulled oats in which only the outermost hull or chaff has been removed. Use as a cereal. Also use as a filler for other flours. *How to Use:* Rolled oats (hulled and flattened) may be used as a breakfast cereal or added to other flours. Steel cut oats can be used to make "porridge," a delicious oatmeal.

HOW TO SLIMFAST WITH WHOLE GRAIN BREADS

Begin by eliminating refined or processed grains and any breads or cakes made with such devitalized flours. Then replace with whole grains for both breads as well as cereals. When you eat these whole grain breads, the bran-fiber content creates an unusual but effective Slimfasting process:

When your digestive system receives the bran-fiber from ingested breads, cakes, pastries or cereals, it reacts by speeding up the metabolic process. The carbohydrate content of bran-fiber is unavailable and indigestible and is NOT absorbed by the system as it energizes the enzymatic function to create speeded-up metabolism of available carbohydrates, calories and fats. This explains why you can Slimfast and lose weight on a bran-fiber bread program. Bran-fiber is not absorbed since it is indigestible as roughage or cellulose. It acts to catalyze other metabolic functions and then passes out of your system. All the time, it satisfies your desire for tasty, wholesome breads, cakes, pastries, cereals—while it slims you down!

Whole grain breads and pastries that are made solely with unbleached, undegerminated, unbolted grains are prime sources of bran-fiber. This miracle nutrient speeds up the transit time of ingested food so that calories (and weight) have little opportunity to be extracted. Therefore, you can have your cake and eat it, too—if it's made of whole grains!

EASY "SEAT-SLIMMING" HIGH FIBER FAST PROGRAM

Louise G. wanted to lose weight *fast* and *forever.* She had a spreading "seat." Her scales showed she was about 15 pounds overweight . . . and then some! She knew she was the victim of an "uncontrollable appetite." She needed something that would nip her appetite in the bud while it slimmed her down. So she turned to an amazingly simple two-day high fiber fast program.

First Day: Louise G. could drink all the fruit and vegetable juices she wanted but she would have to add at least two heaping tablespoons of unprocessed bran to each 8 or 10 ounce glass of juice. *Benefit:* The enzymes in the juice swelled up the particles of the bran into a form of cellulose-roughage within the digestive tract. This created a feeling of "fullness" and appetite satisfaction. Louise G. found she did not care to eat much of anything during this first day.

Second Day: Louise G. could have whole grain cereal with bran and skim milk for breakfast; she could have all the fruit or vegetable salads she wanted throughout the day if she sprinkled some bran and lemon juice for dressing on each one. She could enjoy several slices of whole grain bread with a dab of oil. Dinnertime, Louise G. indulged in breaded veal cutlets or chicken. That's right—breaded— but instead of bread, she used *bran* as the breading. At night, she drank a simple Bran Broth prepared by adding one tablespoon of bran to boiled water containing a bouillon cube. *Benefit:* The use of bran acted as an appetite depressant. Furthermore, the act of having to chew the bran in the cereal or with a salad or as bread or with the meat, gave her an "oral gratification" that acted as a natural control for her previously uncontrollable appetite.

Loses 15 Pounds, Slims Seat. This easy two-day high fiber fast program revitalized her digestive system so that pepped-up metabolism caused the loss of 15 unwanted pounds. Her "seat" was slimmed down. She was now a trim-slim youngish looking woman. To *maintain* her new slim 112 pound weight, Louise G. includes bran as often as she can with her meals and beverages. She calls bran an "all-natural reducing pill!"

FIVE CENTS A DAY KEEPS THE POUNDS AWAY

Plan to take 6 tablespoons of bran daily. *Begin* each of your three meals with 2 tablespoons of bran. This acts as a natural appetite-depressant. Speedily ingested, bran swells up into roughage-cellulose to speed up intestinal transit time so that food leaves the body much more quickly, before calories-carbohydrates-fats can be transformed into excess weight. A simple high fiber fast program is to add 2 tablespoons of bran to any available pure juice (without sugar) and drink it before a meal. Divided up three times daily, you'll soon have a reduced appetite and a reduced body even though you continue eating your favorite foods. Just 5¢ a day (approximate cost of 6 tablespoons of natural and unprocessed bran) can help keep your pounds away . . . permanently!

IN A NUTSHELL

1. Food fiber, also known as roughage or cellulose, creates a "time release" reaction that satisfies your hunger, soothes your appetite.

2. Enjoy 10 different weight-losing benefits on a high fiber fast.

3. Rose D. went on an HFF and lost 39 pounds and unsightly inches, almost overnight. No hunger pangs, no constipation, no starving.

4. Bran is a 5¢ food that is worth a million dollars in results. It's easy to use bran in daily menu planning.

5. Nicholas Z. lost weight on an HFF meat and potatoes Slimfasting program.

6. Slimfast with whole grain bread and products made from these grains.

7. Louise G. lost weight fast and forever on a "seat-slimming" high fiber fast program.

8. Just five cents a day helps keep the pounds away—permanently!

Chapter Eight

Slimfasting Tricks and Tips
to Curb Hunger Pangs
and Control Appetite

Pounds and inches will roll off during any Slimfasting program if you follow a variety of different little methods that curb hunger pangs and help control your appetite. You need to establish a new pattern of eating which will help keep you slim for all of your life. To prevent the recurrence of overweight, follow as many of these mini-Slimfasting tricks as possible.

1. Confine eating to your table. Your Slimfasting program will create more efficient metabolism and *autolysis* if you eat solely at your table rather than in different places.

2. Keep a record of what you eat. This will tell you if you have eaten too much of the wrong foods and you can then plan to eliminate them.

3. If you are discouraged, then stand in front of a mirror without clothes. Take a good, long critical look at yourself. This will renew your faith in continuing your Slimfasting program until you see slimming results.

4. On any Slimfasting program, do *not* eat while watching television or reading. This tends to distract your concentration on your food and your metabolic responses become sluggish.

5. Do your restricted foods lack taste appeal? This problem was solved by food-loving Robert H., who seasons all of his limited foods with spices, herbs, apple cider vinegar or *tart* fruit juices. This helps displace his pound-gaining passion for fats and other high calorie dressings. Robert H. slims down on a simple program of (for example) fresh raw vegetables that he seasons lavishly with these spices and herbs and then drenches with lemon or lime juice. It turns simple foods into sumptuous banquets. He loses pound after pound with no hunger pangs and with no runaway appetite, getting down to his normal weight in about three weeks.

6. To soothe stomach rumbles, try a coffee substitute such as Postum or any herb tea. Use a dab of honey. Helps soothe the urge to eat, too.

7. Alert your metabolism to help give you a feeling of stomach content with regular exercise. Bicycle ride whenever you can. The activity burns up calories and also helps take your mind off your appetite. Walk as often as is comfortably possible.

8. Start off each meal with a glass of plain water or a vegetable juice. It helps put a natural control on your hunger.

9. Snack, if you must—but use fresh vegetables or crunchy fruits. You'll have hunger satiation and controlled appetite.

10. On a Slimfasting program that calls for a meat food, select lean poultry such as chicken or turkey and lean fish, instead of red meats which may be too high in fat for your metabolism to accommodate. Poultry and fish fill you up but do not fatten you out!

11. As often as is comfortably possible, walk up and down the stairs instead of using the elevator. This alerts your respiratory-circulatory systems which oxygenate your internal organs and soothe stomach rumbles.

12. Weigh yourself daily. This will tell you how much progress you are making, or not making. It should help give you an incentive to continue with your Slimfasting program.

13. You'll soothe any desire to eat if you will drink a glass of skim milk. Drink very slowly. Try it through a straw for more satisfaction and appetite control.

14. To give yourself a feeling of "comfortable fullness," increase your intake of roughage. Include whole grains, whole wheat, raw vegetables. This trick helped formerly fat Grace J. lose as much as eight inches from her waistline and trim about fifteen pounds off her body during a Slimfasting program. Grace J. was always plagued by the agonizing stomach rumbles familiar to most reducers; she would "cheat" on her Slimfasting and stuff herself, thereby upsetting her metabolism and halting the weight loss. So Grace J. tried a simple trick. Whenever she felt hungry with the agonizing hunger pangs, she would prepare a cup of boiled water into which she stirred one tablespoon of bran and, if she desired them, a few tablespoons of chopped raw vegetables. The steam helped soften the vegetables so that when she *ate* this all-natural hunger-ease tonic, she felt immediate "fullness" and appetite control. The globules of the bran and vegetables swelled up in her digestive system and she always felt that she had eaten a complete meal. It was her solution to annoying hunger pangs. She was thereby able to lose over eight inches from her waistline and more than fifteen pounds from her body. It made Slimfasting a pleasant joy.

15.   Keep yourself active and occupied during Slimfasting. Get your mind off food. Either work or a hobby is helpful as a form of sublimation so that food is not on your mind.

16.   If you do get the urge to slide off your program, then do something pleasant and luxurious for yourself. Pamper yourself with a long and perfumed bath. Do your fingernails. Give yourself a facial. Put on some of your nicest clothes and go for a window shopping spree. See a movie or other theatrical event. Take a nice walk in a park. *The point is to treat yourself very good so that this self-indulgence will compensate for avoided foods.*

17.   When you set your table for any Slimfasting program, make it look attractive. Use your best napkins, silverware, tablecloth, vase of flowers. It makes Slimfasting a feast, even with modified foods.

18.   During Slimfasting, try to avoid unnecessary food shopping. But if you must go into a food market, do so on a "full" stomach to ease the urge to buy snack and weight-causing foods. Fill up with a plate of diced raw vegetables and radishes, garnished with a dollop of skim milk cottage cheese or drenched with lemon and lime juice. This fills you up and eases the urge to buy and eat unnecessary foods.

19.   If you have a tendency to overeat during Slimfasting, it may help to eat with others on a similar program. This type of "group therapy" bolsters your self-confidence and it is less likely that you will slide off your Slimfasting program.

20.   As you eat your allotted foods, do so very slowly to give yourself oral satisfaction. (Another benefit is that slow chewing triggers off a rich treasure of digestive juices to flow and create better metabolism and burning of foods.) Think about the flavors, textures, fragrances.

21.   Seized with a craving for chocolate eclairs or seven layer cake? Get yourself a huge portion of these weight-gaining foods. Put the food on a plate in front of you. Ask yourself if indulgence is worth the added pounds and inches. Then *take one bite* of the chocolate delight. Chew very thoroughly. Continue chewing and chewing the bite until it is liquefied. By maximizing the emotional effect of each bite, you will help reduce your urge to eat this calorie-fat laden food. Many Slimfasters find that just two bites help ease and erase the gnawing urge for the forbidden food.

22.   For a tasty beverage that is nourishing as well as appetite-satisfying, try beef, chicken or vegetable bouillon with one tablespoon of natural bran per average-sized bowl. Only 10 to 20 calories per serving. It's the "safe" snack during a Slimfasting program.

23. Perk up the taste of hot or cold coffee substitute such as Postum or herb tea with a dash of cinnamon. This eliminates the need for sugar.

24. "Cheat" on your Slimfasting program by enjoying a quick snack of sugar-free gelatin dessert. Good source of protein but almost void of calories. *Tip:* Whip sugar-free gelatin desserts when they are half gelled, then refrigerate until they are firm. Whipped, they appear to give you more filling satisfaction.

25. To ease the hunger urge, keep a container of unsweetened ice tea in your refrigerator. When the eating desire strikes, pour yourself a glass. Add a twist of orange peel and then sip slowly. For a pleasant tang that takes away the appetite, try lime or lemon peel in the iced tea.

26. At all times, keep your refrigerator filled with crisp cut-up vegetables. Try green pepper, zucchini, celery, carrots, cauliflower, radishes as well as salad greens and all forms of cabbage including savoy and Chinese. Nibble and chew and feel filled up while Slimfasting.

27. Love to drink milk shakes? So does formerly-fat Allan I. who was literally raised on milk shakes and ice cream sodas. They had made him more than 50 pounds overweight by the time he was in his early twenties. He slimmed down on various Slimfasting programs. But he still indulges in "forbidden" milk shakes with very few calories. Here is how to make the same milk shake that Allan I. enjoys. In a blender container at high speed, blend until smooth 1/2 cup cold water, 1/3 cup nonfat dry milk powder, 7 or 8 ice cubes, 1/2 teaspoon honey and 1 teaspoon vanilla extract. Whizz. Then enjoy this "forbidden" milk shake that gives you all the taste of the real thing with negligible weighty factors. This milk shake is a regular with formerly fat Allan I. who lost more than 50 pounds on Slimfasting, even while drinking this beverage.

28. Fill up on a tomato juice cocktail. Serve fresh tomato juice with a twist of lemon peel, and ice cubes for more of a filling reaction.

29. If your Slimfasting program calls for one major meal, then take it earlier in the day. This gives your body more time to digest and burn off calories. This will also help ease prolonged hunger pains since the process of metabolism helps keep you satisfied.

30. If you find yourself ravenously hungry, train yourself not to eat for 30 minutes. Many Slimfasting folks find that this obsessive urge to eat will diminish greatly if they can hold out for a little while.

31. Avoid contact with overweight friends who do not want to reduce. They make you feel hungry. They may also discourage you, so try to keep away from them until you're slim.

32.   As a substitute for food, try listening to music. It acts as a natural appetite depressant and will help shield you from thoughts of food. If you feel compelled to go to the refrigerator, make a detour and head for your record player instead. Listen to any gentle music that is *not* the explosive or ear-shattering type which tends to alert your senses and increase your appetite. Classical music is soothing. Listen to it; concentrate on the sound; become immersed in each note. This helps replace the urge to eat.

33.   You're at a party surrounded by many weight-laden foods. You feel the urge to eat. What to do? To begin with, you could avoid partying until you've slimmed down. But if you must go, then stick to any available low-calorie snacks, such as celery stalks or carrot sticks. If possible, bring along some in a plastic bag (assuming none may be available) and munch away freely. Hors d'oeuvres tempting you? Can't resist? Then eat some . . . but compensate by skipping much of everything else, including any main meal.

34.   If you're going to be faced with very severe stress such as a long business or family tour or trip, or any emotional tension, then delay Slimfasting. Otherwise, the combination of metabolic change plus emotional stress may counteract results and cause uncontrollable hunger. *It's better to delay than to begin Slimfasting badly.* One bad start can weaken your resolve for months. Give yourself the best chance possible.

35.   Pinpoint those times when you have the "appetite urge" to eat fattening foods or to slide off your Slimfasting program. For example, do you have hunger pangs just before noon? Or maybe you like to munch in mid-afternoon. Each person is different. *It is your obligation to identify your "hunger hours" and mark them down, giving the specific time.* What to do? When you can anticipate this urge, plan to be out of the house and away from food at that hour. Go jogging. Play golf. Play tennis. Take a long walk in an area where food is not available. Do *anything* you want but get away from food during your "hunger hours."

36.   When you weigh yourself and see the pounds going off, and when you tape measure yourself to see inches going off on Slimfasting, give yourself a little "gift" or present. Buy that lovely shawl that you thought was too expensive. Buy a new hanging plant. Buy that nice vase. Or buy that long-desired tool kit. But do this ONLY if you do not cheat. This "reward system" should be followed weekly as a means of bolstering your self-control over appetite and hunger.

37.   You may become the victim of "diet temper." This was the problem of Jacqueline R. Any reducing program would make her

grouchy and surly with churning hunger pains. Jacqueline solved "diet temper" on her Slimfasting program with this simple method: whenever she felt waves of hunger, she would go right to the bedroom, close the door and lie down on her bed. She would punch her pillow! She would hit it with every bit of strength she had. If Jacqueline R. felt especially temperamental because of hunger pains, she would yell out loud, "I don't like this diet!" and keep hitting the pillow. It took about 15 minutes and it worked to soothe and relax her feelings of hunger. This punching-yelling scheme helped release her feelings, helped soothe the intensity of her emotions and relaxed her "diet temper." When she left the bedroom, she felt better and eagerly looked forward to continuation of her Slimfasting program.

38.   To divert your attention from a growling stomach, try massage. The kneading and stroking help transfer your focussed thoughts from foods to other parts of your body. You could begin a self-massage program this way: Sprinkle some body oil such as baby lotion or ordinary vegetable oil all over yourself. Then start to rub yourself all over. Use simple stroking, kneading, pulling, tapping strokes. Self-massage yourself on your legs, thighs, stomach, hips, upper arms and shoulders and every other body part that is comfortable to reach. This eases your thoughts and feelings about food and you'll find yourself feeling very relaxed and "de-hungrified!"

39.   A warm leisurely soak in a perfumed tub is most relaxing. The water on the body helps to "seal" in the efforts of metabolism and appears to increase them. After a 20 minute soak, take a quick needle-spray cool shower, rub dry with a thick Turkish towel and then relax in bed. You'll find that gnawing hunger of the mind and/or body is now pampered and contented.

40.   Breathing is a good way to send a stream of fresh cell- and tissue-feeding oxygen throughout your body. It is also a good way to take the edge off your appetite. Take a deep breath, count to ten, then breathe out. As you do this, visualize all tensions leaving your body. Concentrate on "air washing" yourself of all anxieties, frustrations and problems in one big whoosh! Repeat this simple breathing exercise a number of times during the day and you should feel comfortable and, again, "de-hungrified!"

41.   On a Slimfasting program, if you just love pasta, or if you are an ice cream addict, or if you go into ecstasies over syrup-topped cheese cake, you need not cut out these foods altogether. Instead, *cut down on them.* Reason? Lifelong addiction to certain foods may cause digestive rebellion when there is denial. On Slimfasting, you may omit them for a week, but then you'll end up going wild in frustration

and gobbling up these heavy, fattening favorites. So cut down on portions if you're frothing at the mouth for your delicious taboos. Eat *very small portions* when the uncontrollable urge hits you. This eases your urge. The "law of the minimum" applies here. A little bit can go a long way. You'll taper off gradually and soon may have no stomach rumbles at all, when these taboo foods are permanently eliminated.

42.   The urge to nibble something sweet is often a mental situation. If you have this urge, reach for a very thin slice of fresh lemon or lime. *Benefit:* The tart taste of the slice will soothe your taste buds and help eliminate that craving for sweets entirely. It's the easy way to enjoy your Slimfasting without a "sweet appetite" urge.

43.   When preparing foods for your Slimfasting program, make only as much as the schedule calls for. That way, you won't be tempted to overeat. What you do *not* see before you, will *not* excite your appetite.

44.   At times, you may awaken in the night and feel the urge for a "midnight raid" on the refrigerator. The vision of a thick slice of chocolate cake will start your stomach churning. Prepare yourself in advance. Hook up an alarm system, buzzer or bells to the refrigerator, so when you open the door in the middle of the night, the alarm will go off. This alerts you to the risk of overeating. It should help soothe your urge, give you a laugh and help you return to bed. At most, it will awaken others in your home and their protests may make you forget your hunger real quick.

45.   Throughout the day, drink lots and lots of water. It is the best way to fill you up without adding weight. Water also promotes the cleansing of impurities and fat-causing waste materials from your body. Instead of food, try drinking water!

46.   If you feel discouraged, then look through any of the fashion magazines featuring the beautiful models and film stars of the world. Visualize yourself being as slim and attractive as they are. Tell yourself that with Slimfasting you can nip the hunger-appetite urge in the bud and open the doorway to a new "forever slim" figure that is the picture of youthful health.

Select any Slimfasting program in this book. Then follow it with hope and anticipation. Prepare yourself for occasional backsliding. Use any or as many of these Slimfasting tricks and tips that will help curb your hunger pangs and soothe your appetite. Be the master of your Slimfasting program and you will take off pounds and inches and keep them off permanently!

SPECIAL POINTS

1. Ease the problem of gnawing hunger pangs and uncontrollable appetite with any of the 46 tricks and tips presented herewith.

2. Robert H. uses spices, herbs, apple cider vinegar or tart fruit juice as seasonings to put zest and gourmet taste into everyday foods. It makes Slimfasting a feast of weight-losing results.

3. Grace J. uses an all-natural hunger-ease tonic to give her immediate "fullness" and appetite control with almost no calories.

4. Allan I. lost over 50 pounds on Slimfasting while he continued to enjoy a "forbidden" milk shake that soothed his appetite as weight rolled off.

5. Jacqueline R. conquered her "diet temper" by hitting the pillow and yelling at it for 15 minutes.

6. You can "de-hungrify" yourself and Slimfast your way to a permanently lean and healthy figure.

Chapter Nine

How to Chew Your Calories
and Lose Weight with Slimfasting

Whether you tip your scales by five pounds or by fifty pounds, you can shed excess weight through a "no fuss" calorie control Slimfasting program.

CALORIES ARE NOT ALL ALIKE

A Slimfasting program that emphasizes *chewy foods high in calories* can help you lose more weight than a program that suggests cutting down on calories alone. Calorie containing foods that require you to chew and chew can help give you a feeling of appetite satisfaction, stomach contentment and less weight than those calorie containing foods that you eat and swallow with minimum eating effort. Calories are not all alike and here is the reason:

A broiled steak, a chunk of coarse whole grain black bread, a succulent ear of whole-kernel corn, a honey-sweetened pastry made with thick whole grains will require a great deal of chewing. When you eat these "chewy" caloric foods, your body will receive fewer calories than you swallow. Calories from "chewy" foods create stronger digestive juices and enzymes which prompt more thorough assimilation of the calories.

"CHEWY" FOODS VS. REFINED FOODS

Foods that require chewing will put on less weight than those refined foods that are easily gulped down, *even though both may have the same amount of calories.* Your easy and tasty Slimfasting program need emphasize *only* those foods that require thorough chewing and you can lose weight while you enjoy most of your favorite but "chewy" meals. Here is the reason why this Slimfasting "chewy" food program can lose pounds and inches very quickly while you delight in many caloric foods:

The amount of calories your body receives from eaten food is determined by the length of time this food remains in your digestive system. Weight gain is influenced by the speed with which digestive juices (enzymes) are able to get to and metabolize the food you have swallowed. It takes time to fully metabolize every calorie. "Chewy" or "fibrous" foods pass through your system speedily because the very act of chewing sent forth a shower of enzymes that broke down those foods into nutrients that are absorbable. The amount of calories you received from this swift-passing food is less than that which the food contained.

Refined foods (such as bleached white bread, pre-cooked frozen dinners, canned foods) require almost *no* chewing. Therefore, your bloodstream instantly takes up the nutrients and these include the heavy calories that put on weight. Refined, processed and fiber-free foods offer empty or naked calories and carbohydrates. Refined foods have been stripped of natural bulk that would require chewing. The end result is that the food you eat is made up of calories and carbohydrates. Passing through your system without the need for chewing, these refined foods are seized by the bloodstream which absorbs the weight-causing calories and carbohydrates.

A Slimfasting "Chewy" Program
Melts Stubborn Pounds

Charles O'C. needed to lose some 45 pounds. His doctor told Charles he had a choice of either giving up most of his favorite foods or running the risk of ill health through the constantly growing weight and waistline. So Charles O'C. was glad to hear of a Slimfasting program that would let him eat many of his favorite foods and would also slim him down. Here is the Slimfasting "Chewy" Program that helped him lose more than 45 of his stubborn pounds:

1. All foods had to be fresh, natural and as free from refinement as possible.

2. Grain foods had to be made from whole grains, nonprocessed, high in fiber and bulk. Breakfast cereals could be buckwheat, granola, oatmeal, French toast—provided that the source was chewy and bulk-producing.

3. He could indulge in reduced but satisfying portions of his favorite pastries and an occasional cake slice but they had to be made from unbleached flour, high in fiber and bulk.

4. Main dish foods such as meat could be enjoyed but they had to be from a natural source. That is, a steak, a lamb chop, a casserole, a stew, a goulash could be enjoyed but all ingredients had to be fresh and natural. No precooked canned, frozen, dehydrated ingredients of any sort.

5. He could have lots of raw fruits and vegetables but these
    were to be chewed thoroughly.

POUND AFTER POUND DISAPPEARS

Under this delicious and "chewy" good Slimfasting program, Charles O'C. could enjoy most of his beloved foods and still lose weight. The scales told him that pound after pound just disappeared until after four months, he had finally lost more than the 45 stubborn pounds. He had a neat 32 inch waistline, a youthful physique. He felt good and glad all over, thanks to a Slimfasting program that required only one basic rule: *all foods had to be chewed and as natural as possible.*

Why "Chewy" Foods Are Lower in Calories

When you chew fibrous or bulk-containing foods (including a once-forbidden pastry that should be prepared from whole grains and natural products), you immediately alert a metabolic reaction in your system.

Your metabolism works swiftly to burn up the calories and transforms them so that they can be used for *energy* and *not* stored as weight. The chewing process alerts this metabolic reaction.

Conversely, refined foods that require no chewing do *not* call for metabolic digestion. Therefore, the calories from refined foods are speedily absorbed by the bloodstream and this causes weight gain.

The very act of food-burning causes a form of natural weight loss. Compare it to the burning of a fire. *Just as fuel is oxidized or burned to produce energy, in each body cell step-by-step reactions systematically break down large caloric molecules which are then oxidized to release small sources of energy. It is this internal method of cellular oxidation that creates internal combustion.* Calories will not be stored too excessively because of this metabolic reaction.

Chewing acts as the sparkplug to create this caloric-breakdown and dispersion response. Therefore, foods that require healthy chewing will put on much less weight than refined and pre-cooked foods that require no chewing.

HOW TO BEGIN YOUR SLIMFASTING
CALORIE CONTROL PROGRAM

Decide how many calories you need daily. Decide the weight level you wish to achieve. Write it down. Daily, write down how many pounds you lose. Be honest with yourself if you want to succeed.

About Calories. Calories are units of energy found in almost all foods.

Calories in Fat. There are approximately 3500 calories in each stored pound of fat. So if you lose as little as one pound a week, consume 500 fewer calories each day than if you were already at your desired weight.

CALCULATING YOUR CALORIE CONTROL PROGRAM

Here's how to do it:

150	pounds desired weight
x15	calories
2250	calories needed to maintain desired weight
-500	calories daily to lose one pound per week
1750	maximum daily calories

OR, if you want to lose two pounds each week. . .

150	pounds desired weight
x15	calories
2250	calories needed to maintain desired weight
-1000	calories daily to lose two pounds per week
1250	maximum daily calories

Based upon your desired weight goal and your age, how many calories can you enjoy daily? The chart in Figure 9-1 is your guideline.

A Calorie-Chewing Slimfasting
Program for "Impossible Overweight"

As an active housewife, part-time department store supervisor and active clubwoman, Barbara Q. had no time for involved reducing programs. Yet she had to get rid of her "impossible overweight."

Not only did she have more than 37 unwanted, undesirable, unattractive pounds, but she was developing an unsightly double chin and heavy jowls. She had thick "inches" on her hips and thighs. She looked and felt much older than her 45 years.

A look in the mirror told her she needed to lose weight fast, or continue losing her attractiveness. Other diets worked but they left her often feeling weak, hungry and temperamental. She wanted to lose weight but still feel energetic, satisfied, cheerful. So it was that she tried an easy *Calorie-Chewing Slimfasting Program:*

Set Calorie and Weight Goals. Barbara Q. decided how many calories she would eat daily in order to slim down to her desired and agreed upon weight.

DAILY MAINTENANCE CALORIES

	Desired Weight	18-35 years	35-55 years	55-75 years
WOMEN	99	1700	1500	1300
	110	1850	1650	1400
	121	2000	1750	1550
	128	2100	1900	1600
	132	2150	1950	1650
	143	2300	2050	1800
	154	2400	2150	1850
	165	2550	2300	1950
MEN	110	2200	1950	1650
	121	2400	2150	1850
	132	2550	2300	1950
	143	2700	2400	2050
	154	2900	2600	2200
	165	3100	2800	2400
	176	3250	2950	2500
	187	3300	3100	2600

Note: Calorie counts are based on moderate activity. If your life is very active, add calories. If your life is very sedentary, subtract calories.

Figure 9-1

Select Lower-Calorie Foods. From a calorie count list (as in this chapter) she selected a wide variety of foods that would meet her daily needs.

Keep Records. Daily, she would weigh herself and keep a record of how much she lost.

Eat Chewy Foods Only. Barbara Q. could eat a variety of most of her favorite foods, provided they required lots of healthy and normal chewing. She could eat a slice of pizza or chunk of bread provided it was made of whole grains, with as few refined ingredients as possible. She could eat some beef stew, steak, even a piece of cake, but again, the ingredients were to be natural and the food had to require much chewing.

CUT DOWN, CUT OUT REFINED-PROCESSED-PRECOOKED FOODS

Barbara Q. gradually cut down her eating of refined-processed-precooked foods, then cut them out entirely. She found it was easy when natural and chewy foods replaced the desire for processed foods. *Benefits:* Chewy foods promote metabolic reaction to slim down the bulging fat cells. During overweight, normal muscle-fibre cells become engorged and transformed into fat cells. During a chewy Slimfasting program, metabolism is increased so that caloric burning is able to "attack" the dormant fat cells, loosen and "burn up" the accumulations, then slim them down into normal muscle-fibre cells. This is possible with wholesome and natural foods that require chewing, the action that alerts the cell-slimming response.

FROM "IMPOSSIBLE" TO "POSSIBLE" SLIMMING

Daily, Barbara Q. weighed herself. She saw how pounds and inches were actually melting right out of her body. The "impossible" dream was now "possible" slimming, as more than 37 pounds vanished from her body. The inches on her hips melted away. Soon, Barbara Q. was a slim-trim, youngish looking girl. Her face was firm. Her hips were lean. She looked, felt and acted cheerfully young. Her overweight was gone . . . forever!

THE "CELL-SLIMMING" FACTOR IN CALORIE-CHEWING SLIMFASTING

Calorie-containing foods that require chewing can create a "cell-slimming" reaction that will melt away pounds and shrink down inches! Foods that are chewed create a form of spontaneous combustion. This "heat" powers your digestive system to metabolize and then *transform* accumulated fat in the cells into small amounts of carbohydrates. The digestive system now seizes these carbohydrates, uses them as a form of self-energy to break down body fat into essential fatty acids that give you vitality during Slimfasting. Cellular fat is also broken down, then it is "melted" away.

CELLS WASHED WITH WATER REMOVAL

Calorie-chewing will then activate a sluggish digestive enzyme system so that stored up intercellular water can be discharged. This serves a double-benefit. The metabolic reaction causes water to wash out of the cells to (1) slim them down and (2) wash them of toxic wastes. The result is that the fat cells are broken down and transformed into healthy muscle-fibre. It is the healthy way to lose weight.

AVOID REFINED, PROCESSED, PACKAGED FOODS

These are pre-cooked and even pre-digested foods. They have been refined, processed, frozen and packaged. They require almost no chewing! They are also heavily laden with salt. When they enter your system, the salt causes a gathering of water. Salt will absorb water and cause cells to become heavy. Furthermore, such refined foods are high in calories and carbohydrates. They require almost NO chewing. Any "chewing" must be done by your digestive system. This means that the salt and other preservatives are taken out and they become engorged with water and will cause weight gain.

IN BRIEF:

The more you chew your food, the shorter it remains in your system during the "transit-time" so that salt and calories do not remain too long in your body. The less you chew your food, the longer it remains in your system during the "transit-time" so that salt and calories accumulate and you gain weight.

The key to a calorie-controlled Slimfasting program is, *firstly,* selecting lower calorie foods and *secondly,* selecting only those that require much chewing. Here it is, at-a-glance:

Longer chewing = shorter "transit-time" = fewer calories

Shorter chewing = longer "transit-time" = more calories

OFFICIAL U.S. GOVERNMENT[1] RECOMMENDATIONS FOR CALORIE CONTROL

To help you Slimfast on a calorie-control program, here are the official U.S. Government's recommendations plus food portion counts:

"To control your weight, you will need to control the amount of energy (the number of calories) you get from food, and the amount of energy you use up in exercise and normal activity.

"Whether you gain weight, lose weight or stay the same depends on how well you balance the calories furnished by the foods you eat against the calories your body uses. If your food furnishes more

---

[1]*Calories And Weight,* U.S. Department of Agriculture, Information Bulletin No. 364, June, 1974, Washington, D.C.

calories than you use, you gain weight. It if furnishes fewer, you lose. If it furnishes just enough, your weight should stay about the same.

"For every 3500 extra calories you get and do not use, you gain about 1 pound of weight. This pound represents stored food energy in the form of fat. To lose excess fat you have to somehow use up stored energy. You can:

"Eat less food (fewer calories), to force your body to draw energy from its stored fat.

"Increase your activity, to use up more energy.

"Do both. Many dieters find a combination of eating less food and getting more exercise the best way to lose weight.

"Remember, the weight that is best for you in your mid-twenties is best for you in later years, too."

TABLE OF CALORIES

Calorie values given for foods in the following tables do not include calories from added fat, sugar, sauce, or dressing—unless such items are included in the listing. Cup measure refers to a standard 8-ounce measuring cup, unless otherwise stated. Foods are listed in the following groups:

- Beverages (carbonated and alcoholic; fruit drinks)
- Bread and cereal group
- Desserts and other sweets
- Fats, oils, and related products (includes salad dressings)
- Meat group (includes fish, eggs, nuts, dry beans and peas)
- Milk group (includes cheeses, milk desserts)
- Snacks and other "extras"
- Soups
- Vegetable-fruit group (includes fruit juices)

BEVERAGES
[Not including milk and fruit juices]

		Calories
Carbonated beverages:		
Cola-type	8-ounce glass	95
	12-ounce can or bottle . . .	145
Fruit flavors, 10-13%	8-ounce glass	115
sugar.	12-ounce can or bottle . . .	170
Ginger ale.	8-ounce glass	75
	12-ounce can or bottle . .	115
Root beer	8-ounce glass	100
	12-ounce can or bottle . . .	150

(Check the label of "low-calorie" drinks for the number of calories provided.)

		Calories
Alcoholic beverages:		
Beer, 3-6% alcohol	8-ounce glass	100
	12-ounce can or bottle . . .	150
Whiskey, gin, rum, vodka:		
80-proof	1 1/2-ounce jigger	95
86-proof	1 1/2-ounce jigger	105
90-proof	1 1/2-ounce jigger	110
100-proof	1 1/2-ounce jigger	125
Wines:		
Table wines	3 1/2-ounce glass	85
(Chablis, claret, Rhine wine, sauterne, etc.).		
Dessert wines	3 1/2-ounce glass	140
(muscatel, port, sherry, Tokay, etc.).		
Fruit drinks:		
Apricot nectar	1/2 cup	70
Cranberry juice cocktail. .	1/2 cup	80
Grape drink	1/2 cup	70
Lemonade, frozen concentrate, sweetened, ready-to-serve.	1/2 cup	55
Orange juice-apricot juice drink	1/2 cup	60
Peach nectar	1/2 cup	60
Pear nectar	1/2 cup	65
Pineapple juice-grapefruit juice drink.	1/2 cup.	70
Pineapple juice-orange juice drink.	1/2 cup	70

BREAD AND CEREAL GROUP

Bread:		
Cracked wheat	1 slice, 18 slices per pound loaf.	65
Raisin	1 slice, 18 slices per pound loaf.	65
Rye	1 slice, 18 slices per pound loaf.	60
White:		
Soft crumb:		
Regular slice	1 slice, 18 slices per pound loaf.	70
Thin slice	1 slice, 22 slices per pound loaf.	55
Firm crumb	1 slice, 20 slices per pound loaf.	65
Whole wheat:		
Soft crumb	1 slice, 16 slices per pound loaf.	65
Firm crumb	1 slice, 18 slices per pound loaf.	60
Biscuits, muffins, rolls:		
Baking powder biscuit:		
Home recipe	2-inch-diameter biscuit . . .	105
Mix	2-inch-diameter biscuit . . .	90
Muffins:		
Plain	3-inch-diameter muffin . . .	120
Blueberry	2 3/8-inch-diameter muffin. .	110
Bran	2 5/8-inch-diameter muffin. .	105
Corn.	2 3/8-inch-diameter muffin. .	125

Calories

Rolls:
Danish pastry, plain . . .	4 1/2-inch-diameter	275
Hanburger or frankfurter .	1 roll (16 per pound) . . .	120
Hard, round or rectangular .	1 roll (9 per pound)	155
Plain, pan	1 roll (16 per pound) . . .	85
Sweet, pan	1 roll (11 per pound) . . .	135

Other flour-based foods:

Cakes, cookies, pies . . . . . (See Desserts.)

Crackers:
Butter	About 2-inch-diameter cracker.	15
Cheese	About 2-inch-diameter cracker.	15
Graham	Two, 2 1/2-inches square . .	55
Matzoth	6-inch-diameter piece . . .	80
Oyster	10	35
Pilot	1	75
Rye	Two, 1 7/8 x 3 1/2 inches . .	45
Saltines	Four, 1 7/8 inches square . .	50

Doughnuts:
Cake-type, plain	3 1/4-inch-diameter (1 1/2 ounces).	165
Yeast-leavened, raised . .	3 3/4-inch-diameter (1 1/2 ounces).	175

Pancakes (griddle cakes):
Wheat (home recipe or mix)	4-inch cake	60
Buckwheat (with buckwheat pancake mix). . . .	4-inch cake	55

Pizza, plain cheese . . . . 5 1/3-inch sector of 13 3/4-inch pie. 155

Pretzels:
Dutch, twisted	1	60
Stick	5 regular (3 1/8 inches long) or 10 small (2 1/4 inches long).	10

Spoonbread	1/2 cup	235
Waffles	7-inch waffle	210

Breakfast cereals:
Bran flakes (40% bran) . . .	1 ounce (about 4/5 cup) . .	85
Bran flakes with raisins . . .	1 ounce (about 3/5 cup) . .	80
Corn, puffed, presweetened .	1 ounce (about 1 cup) . . .	115
Corn, shredded	1 ounce (about 1 1/6 cups). .	110
Corn flakes	1 ounce (about 1 1/6 cups). .	110
Corn flakes, sugar-coated . .	1 ounce (about 2/3 cup) . .	110
Farina, cooked, quick-cooking .	3/4 cup	80
Oats, puffed	1 ounce (about 1 1/6 cups). .	115
Oats, puffed, sugar-coated . .	1 ounce (about 4/5 cup) . .	115
Oatmeal or rolled oats, cooked.	3/4 cup	100
Rice Flakes	1 ounce (about 1 cup) . . .	110
Rice, puffed	1 ounce (about 2 cups) . . .	115
Rice, puffed, presweetened . .	1 ounce (about 2/3 cup) . .	110
Rice, shredded	1 ounce (about 1 1/8 cups). .	115
Wheat, puffed	1 ounce (about 1 7/8 cups). .	105
Wheat, puffed, presweetened. .	1 ounce (about 4/5 cup) . .	105
Wheat, rolled, cooked . . .	3/4 cup	135
Wheat, shredded, plain . . .	1 ounce (1 large biscuit or 1/2 cup bite-size).	100

		Calories
Wheat flakes	1 ounce (about 1 cup)	100
Other grain products:		
Corn grits, degermed, cooked	3/4 cup	95
Macaroni, cooked:		
Plain	3/4 cup	115
With cheese, home recipe	1/2 cup	215
With cheese, canned	1/2 cup	115
Noodles, cooked	3/4 cup	150
Rice, cooked, instant	3/4 cup	135
Spaghetti, cooked:		
Plain	3/4 cup	115
In tomato sauce, with cheese, home recipe.	3/4 cup	195
In tomato sauce, with cheese, canned.	3/4 cup	140
With meat balls, home recipe.	3/4 cup	250
With meat balls, canned.	3/4 cup	195
Wheat germ, toasted	1 tablespoon	25

DESSERTS AND OTHER SWEETS

Cakes:		
Angelcake	2 1/2-inch sector of 9 3/4-inch round cake.	135
Boston cream pie	2 1/8-inch sector of 8-inch round cake.	210
Chocolate cake, with chocolate icing.	1 3/4-inch sector of 9-inch round layer cake.	235
Fruitcake, dark	2 x 1 1/2 x 1/4-inch slice	55
Gingerbread	2 3/4 x 2 3/4 x 1 3/8-inch slice.	175
Plain cake:		
Without icing	3 x 3 x 2-inch slice	315
	2 3/4-inch-diameter cupcake.	115
With chocolate icing.	1 3/4-inch sector of 9-inch round layer cake.	240
	2 3/4-inch-diameter cupcake.	170
Pound cake, old fashioned	3 1/2 x 3 x 1/2-inch slice	140
Sponge cake	1 7/8-inch sector of 9 3/4-inch round cake.	145
Candies:		
Caramels	3 medium (1 ounce)	115
Chocolate creams	2 to 3 pieces (1 ounce), 35 to a pound.	125
Chocolate, milk, sweetened	1-ounce bar	145
Chocolate, milk, sweetened, with almonds.	1-ounce bar	150
Chocolate mints	1 to 2 mints (1 ounce), 20 to a pound.	115
Fondant:		
Candy corn	20 pieces (1 ounce)	105
Mints	Three 1 1/2-inch mints (1 ounce).	105

Calories

Fudge, vanilla or chocolate:

Plain	1 ounce	115
	1-inch cube	85
With nuts	1 ounce	120
	1-inch cube	90
Gumdrops	About 2 1/2 large or 20 small (1 ounce).	100
Hard candy	Three or four 3/4-inch-diameter candy balls (1 ounce).	110
Jellybeans	10 (1 ounce)	105
Marshmallows	4 large	90
Peanut brittle	1 1/2 pieces, 2 1/2 x 1 1/4 x 3/8-inch (1 ounce).	120

Other sweets:

Chocolate:

Bittersweet	1-ounce square	135
Semisweet	1-ounce square	145

Chocolate syrup:

Thin type	1 tablespoon	45
Fudge type	1 tablespoon	60
Cranberry sauce, canned	1 tablespoon	25
Honey	1 tablespoon	65
Jam, preserves	1 tablespoon	55
Jelly, marmalade	1 tablespoon	50
Molasses	1 tablespoon	50
Syrup, table blends	1 tablespoon	55
Sugar, white, granulated, or brown (packed).	1 teaspoon	15

Cookies:

Chocolate chip	2 1/2-inch cooky, 1/2 inch thick	50
Figbar	1 small	50
Sandwich, chocolate or vanilla.	1 3/4-inch cooky, 3/8-inch thick	50
Sugar	2 1/4-inch cooky	35
Vanilla wafer	1 3/4-inch cooky	20

Pies:

Apple	1/8 of 9-inch pie	300
Blueberry	1/8 of 9-inch pie	285
Cherry	1/8 of 9-inch pie	310
Chocolate meringue	1/8 of 9-inch pie	285
Coconut custard	1/8 of 9-inch pie	270
Custard, plain	1/8 of 9-inch pie	250
Lemon meringue	1/8 of 9-inch pie	270
Mince	1/8 of 9-inch pie	320
Peach	1/8 of 9-inch pie	300
Pecan	1/8 of 9-inch pie	430
Pumpkin	1/8 of 9-inch pie	240
Raisin	1/8 of 9-inch pie	320
Rhubarb	1/8 of 9-inch pie	300
Strawberry	1/8 of 9-inch pie	185

Calories

Other desserts:
Apple betty	1/2 cup	160
Bread pudding, with raisins.	1/2 cup	250
Brownie, with nuts	1 3/4 inches square, 7/8-inch thick.	90
Custard, baked	1/2 cup	150
Fruit ice	1/2 cup	125

Gelatin:
Plain	1/2 cup	70
With fruit	1/2 cup	80

Ice cream, plain:
Regular (about 10%fat)	1/2 cup	130
Rich (about 16% fat).	1/2 cup	165

Ice milk:
Hardened	1/2 cup	100
Soft serve	1/2 cup	135
Prune whip	1/2 cup	70

Puddings:
Cornstarch, vanilla	1/2 cup	140
Chocolate, from a mix	1/2 cup	160
Rennet desserts, ready-to-serve.	1/2 cup	115
Tapioca cream	1/2 cup	110
Sherbet	1/2 cup	130

FATS, OILS, AND RELATED PRODUCTS

Butter or margarine	1 pat, 1 inch square, 1/2 inch thick.	35
	1 tablespoon	100
Margarine, whipped	1 pat, 1 1/4 inches squares, 1/3 inch thick.	25
	1 tablespoon	70

Cooking fats:
Vegetable	1 tablespoon	110
Lard	1 tablespoon	115
Peanut butter	(See Meat Group; other high-protein foods.)	

Salad dressings:

Regular:
Blue cheese	1 tablespoon	75
French	1 tablespoon	65
Home-cooked, boiled	1 tablespoon	25
Italian	1 tablespoon	85
Mayonnaise	1 tablespoon	100
Salad dressing, commercial, plain mayonnaise-type).	1 tablespoon	65
Russian	1 tablespoon	75
Thousand Island	1 tablespoon	80

Low calorie:
French	1 tablespoon	15
Italian	1 tablespoon	10
Thousand Island	1 tablespoon	25
Salad oil	1 tablespoon	120

MEAT GROUP

Calories

Beef:
   Beef and vegetable stew:

		Calories
Canned	1 cup	195
Homemade, with lean beef .	1 cup	220
Beef potpie, home prepared, baked.	1/4 of 9-inch-diameter pie . .	385

Chili con carne, canned:

With beans	1/2 cup	170
Without beans . . .	1/2 cup	240
Corned beef, canned . . .	3 ounces	185
Corned beef hash . . .	2/5 cup (3 ounces) . . .	155
Dried beef, chipped . . .	1/3 cup (2 ounces) . . .	115
Dried beef, creamed . .	1/2 cup	190

Hamburger, broiled,
    panbroiled, or sauteed:

Regular	3 ounces	245
Lean	3 ounces	185

Oven roast, cooked, without
    bone:
(Cuts relatively fat, such as rib)

Lean and fat	3 ounces	375
Lean only	3 ounces	205

(Cuts relatively lean, such as round)

Lean and fat	3 ounces	220
Lean only	3 ounces	160

Pot roast, cooked, braised or
    simmered, without bone:

Lean and fat	3 ounces	245
Lean only	3 ounces	165

Steak, broiled, without bone:
(Cuts relatively fat, such as sirloin)

Lean and fat	3 ounces	330
Lean only	3 ounces	175

(Cuts relatively lean, such as round)

Lean and fat	3 ounces	220
Lean only	3 ounces	160
Veal cutlet, broiled, without bone, trimmed.	3 ounces	185
Veal roast, cooked, without bone.	3 ounces	230

Lamb:
   Loin chop, broiled, without
     bone:

Lean and fat	3 ounces	305
Lean only	3 ounces	160

   Leg, roasted, without bone:

Lean and fat	3 ounces	235
Lean only	3 ounces	160

   Shoulder, roasted, without
     bone:

Lean and fat	3 ounces	285
Lean only	3 ounces	175

Calories

Pork:

Bacon, broiled or fried, crisp.	2 thin slices	60
	2 medium slices	85
Bacon, Canadian, cooked . .	One 3 3/8 x 3/16-inch slice .	60

Chop, broiled, without bone:

Lean and fat	3 ounces	335
Lean only	3 ounces	230

Ham, cured, cooked, without bone:

Lean and fat	3 ounces	245
Lean only	3 ounces	160

Roast, loin, cooked, without bone:

Lean and fat	3 ounces	310
Lean only	3 ounces	215

Sausage:

Bologna	2 ounces (2 very thin 4 1/2-inch-diameter slices).	170
Braunschweiger	2 ounces (two 3 1/8-inch-diameter slices).	180

Pork sausage:

Link, cooked . . .	Four 4-inch links (4 ounces, uncooked).	250
Bulk, cooked . . .	Two 3 7/8 x 1/4-inch patties (4 ounces, uncooked).	260
Salami	2 ounces (two 4 1/2-inch-diameter slices).	175
Vienna sausage, canned . . .	2 ounces (3 1/2 sausages) . .	135

Variety and luncheon meats:

Beef heart, braised, trimmed .	3 ounces (4 x 2 1/2-inch piece).	160
Beef liver, fried	3 ounces (6 1/2 x 2 3/8 x 3/8-inch piece).	195
Beef tongue, braised . . .	3 ounces (3 x 2 x 3/8-inch piece).	210
Frankfurter, cooked . . .	1 (8 per pound)	170
Boiled ham	2 ounces (2 very thin 6 1/4 x 4-inch slices).	135
Spiced ham, canned	2 ounces (2 thin 3 x 2-inch slices).	165

Poultry:

Chicken:

Broiled (no skin) . . .	1/4 small broiler	115
Fried	1/2 breast	160
	1 thigh	120
	1 drumstick	90
Canned, meat only . . .	1/2 cup (3 1/2 ounces) . . .	200
Poultry pie, home prepared, baked.	1/4 of 9-inch-diameter pie . .	410

Turkey, roasted (no skin):

Light meat	3 ounces	150
Dark meat	3 ounces	175

Calories

Fish and shellfish:
Bluefish, baked	3 ounces (3 1/2 x 2 x 1/2-inch piece).	135
Clams, shelled:		
Canned	3 medium clams and juice (3 ounces).	45
Raw, meat only	4 medium (3 ounces) . . .	65
Crabmeat, canned or cooked .	1/2 cup (3 ounces)	80
Fish sticks, breaded, cooked, frozen.	Three 4 x 1 x 1/2-inch sticks (3 ounces).	150
Haddock, breaded, fried . .	3 ounces (4 x 2 1/2 x 1/2-inch fillet).	140
Mackerel:		
Broiled with fat	3 ounces (4 x 3 x 1/2-inch piece).	200
Canned	2/5 cup with liquid (3 ounces).	155
Ocean perch, breaded, fried. .	3 ounces (4 x 2 1/2 x 1/2-inch piece.)	195
Oysters, raw, meat only . .	1/2 cup (6 to 10 medium) . .	80
Salmon:		
Broiled or baked . . .	3 ounces	155
Canned, pink	3/5 cup with liquid (3 ounces) .	120
Sardines, canned in oil, drained.	7 medium (3 ounces) . . .	170
Shrimp, canned	27 medium (3 ounces) . . .	100
Tunafish, canned in oil, drained.	1/2 cup (3 ounces)	170

Eggs:
Fried in fat	1 large	100
Hard or soft cooked, "boiled."	1 large	80
Omelet, plain	1 large egg, milk, and fat for cooking.	110
Poached	1 large	80
Scrambled in fat	1 large egg and milk	110

Dry beans and peas:
Baked beans, canned:		
With pork and tomato sauce	1/2 cup	155
With pork and sweet sauce .	1/2 cup	190
Limas, cooked	1/2 cup	130
Red kidney beans, canned or cooked.	1/2 cup, with liquid	110

Nuts:
Almonds	15 (2 tablespoons)	105
Brazil nuts	4-5 large (2 tablespoons). . .	115
Cashews	11-12 medium (2 tablespoons).	100
Coconut, fresh, shredded . .	2 tablespoons	55
Peanuts	2 tablespoons	105
Peanut butter	1 tablespoon	95
Pecans, halves	10 jumbo or 15 large . . .	95
Walnuts:		
Black, chopped	2 tablespoons	100
English or Persian	6-7 halves	80
	2 tablespoons, chopped. . .	105

MILK GROUP

		Calories
Milk:		
Buttermilk	1 cup	90
Condensed, sweetened, undiluted.	1/2 cup	490
Evaporated, undiluted . . .	1/2 cup	175
Partly skimmed, 2% nonfat milk solids added.	1 cup	145
Skim	1 cup	90
Whole	1 cup	160
Cream:		
Half-and-half (milk and cream).	1 tablespoon	20
	1 cup	325
Heavy, whipping	1 tablespoon	55
Light, coffee or table . . .	1 tablespoon	30
Light, whipping	1 tablespoon	45
Sour	1 tablespoon	25
Whipped topping, pressurized .	1 tablespoon	10
Imitation cream products (made with vegetable fat):		
Creamers:		
Liquid (frozen)	1 tablespoon	20
Powdered	1 teaspoon	10
Sour dressing (imitation sour cream) made with nonfat dry milk.	1 tablespoon	20
Whipped topping:		
Pressurized	1 tablespoon	10
Frozen	1 tablespoon	10
Powdered, made with whole milk.	1 tablespoon	10
Yogurt:		
Made from partially skimmed milk.	1 cup	125
Made from whole milk . . .	1 cup	150
Milk beverages:		
Chocolate-flavored drink made with skim milk and 2% added butterfat.	1 cup	190
Chocolate-flavored drink made with whole milk.	1 cup	215
Chocolate, homemade . . .	1 cup	240
Chocolate milkshake . . .	One 12-ounce container . .	515
Cocoa, homemade	1 cup	245
Malted milk	1 cup	245
Milk desserts:		
Custard, baked	1 cup	305
Ice cream:		
Regular (about 10% fat). .	1 cup	255
Rich (about 16% fat). . .	1 cup	330
Ice milk:		
Hardened	1 cup	200
Soft-serve	1 cup	265
Sherbet	1/2 cup	130

Calories

Cheese:

American, process	. . . .	1 ounce	105
		1-inch cube	65
American, process cheese food.		1 tablespoon	45
		1-inch cube	55
American, process cheese spread.		1 tablespoon	40
		1 ounce	80
Blue or roquefort-type	. . .	1 ounce	105
		1-inch cube	65
Camembert		1 wedge of a 4-ounce package containing 3 wedges.	115
Cheddar, natural	. . . . .	1 ounce	115
		1-inch cube	70
		1/2 cup, grated (2 ounces) . .	225
Cottage, creamed	. . . . .	2 tablespoons (1 ounce) . .	30
		1 cup, packed	260
Cottage, uncreamed .	. . . .	2 tablespoons (1 ounce) . .	20
		1 cup, packed	170
Cream		1 ounce	105
		1-inch cube	60
Parmesan, grated	. . . . .	1 tablespoon	25
		1 ounce	130
Swiss, natural	. . . . . .	1 ounce	105
		1-inch cube	55
Swiss, process	. . . . . .	1 ounce	100
		1-inch cube	65

SNACKS AND OTHER "EXTRAS"

Calories

Bouillon cube		1 cube, 1/2-inch	5
Cheese sauce (medium white sauce with 2 tablespoons grated cheese per cup).		1/2 cup	205
Corn chips		1 cup	230
Doughnut:			
Cake-type, plain		3 1/4-inch diameter (1 1/2 ounces).	165
Yeast-leavened, raised . . .		3 3/4-inch diameter (1 1/2 ounces).	175
French fries:			
Fresh		Ten 3 1/2 x 1/4-inch pieces .	215
Frozen		Ten 3 1/2 x 1/4-inch pieces .	170
Gravy		2 tablespoons	35
Hamburger (with roll)		2-ounce patty (about 6 patties per pound of raw meat).	280
Hot dog (with roll)		1 average	290
Olives:			
Green		5 small or 3 large or 2 giant .	15
Ripe		3 small or 2 large	15
Pickles:			
Dill		1 3/4 x 4-inch pickle . . .	15
Sweet		3/4 x 2 1/2-inch pickle . . .	20
Pizza, plain cheese		5 1/3-inch sector of 13 3/4-inch pie.	155

		Calories
Popcorn, large-kernel, popped with oil and salt.	1 cup	40
Potato chips	Ten 1 3/4 x 2 1/2-inch chips	115
Pretzels:		
Dutch, twisted	1	60
Stick	5 regular (3 1/8 inches long) or 10 small (2 1/4 inches long).	10
Tomato catsup or chili sauce	1 tablespoon	15
White sauce, medium (1 cup milk, 2 tablespoons fat, 2 tablespoons flour).	1/2 cup	200

SOUPS

[Canned, condensed, prepared with equal volume of water unless otherwise stated]

		Calories
Bean with pork	1 cup	170
Beef noodle	1 cup	65
Bouillon, broth, or consomme	1 cup	30
Chicken gumbo	1 cup	55
Chicken noodle	1 cup	60
Chicken with rice	1 cup	50
Clam chowder, Manhattan	1 cup	80
Cream of asparagus:		
With water	1 cup	65
With milk	1 cup	145
Cream of chicken:		
With water	1 cup	95
With milk	1 cup	180
Cream of mushroom:		
With water	1 cup	135
With milk	1 cup	215
Minestrone	1 cup	105
Oyster stew (frozen):		
With water	1 cup	120
With milk	1 cup	200
Pea, split	1 cup	145
Tomato:		
With water	1 cup	90
With milk	1 cup	170
Vegetable with beef broth	1 cup	80

VEGETABLE–FRUIT GROUP

		Calories
Vegetables (raw):		
Cabbage, Plain	1/2 cup, shredded, chopped, or sliced.	10
Coleslaw, with mayonnaise.	1/2 cup	85
Coleslaw, with mayonnaise-type salad dressing.	1/2 cup	60
Carrots	7 1/2 x 1 1/8-inch carrot	30
	1/2 cup, grated	25

Calories

Celery	Three 5-inch stalks	10
Chicory	1/2 cup, 1/2-inch pieces	5
Chives	1 tablespoon	Trace
Cucumbers, pared	6 center slices, 1/8 inch thick	5
Endive	1/2 cup, small pieces	5
Lettuce	2 large leaves	5
	1/2 cup, shredded or chopped	5
	1 wedge, 1/6 of head	10

Onions:

Young green	2 medium or 6 small, without tops.	15
	1 tablespoon, chopped	5
Mature	1 tablespoon, chopped	5
Parsley	1 tablespoon, chopped	Trace
Peppers, green	1 ring, 1/4 inch thick	Trace
	1 tablespoon, chopped	Trace
Radishes	5 medium	5
Tomatoes	2 2/5-inch diameter tomato.	20
Turnips	1/2 cup, cubed or sliced	20
Watercress	10 sprigs	5

Vegetables (cooked, canned, or frozen):

Asparagus spears	6 medium or 1/2 cup cut	20

Beans:

Green lima	1/2 cup	90
Snap, green, wax or yellow	1/2 cup	15
Beets	1/2 cup, diced, sliced, or small whole.	30
Beet greens	1/2 cup	15
Broccoli	1/2 cup chopped, or three 4 1/2 to 5-inch stalks.	25
Brussels sprouts	1/2 cup (four 1 1/4 to 1 1/2-inch sprouts).	25
Cabbage	1/2 cup	15
Carrots	1/2 cup	25
Cauliflower	1/2 cup flower buds	15
Celery	1/2 cup, diced	10
Chard	1/2 cup	15
Collards	1/2 cup	25

Corn:

On cob	One 5-inch ear	70
Kernels, drained	1/2 cup	70
Cream-style	1/2 cup	105
Cress, garden	1/2 cup	15
Dandelion greens	1/2 cup	15
Eggplant	1/2 cup, diced	20
Kale	1/2 cup	20
Kohlrabi	1/2 cup	20
Mushrooms, canned	1/2 cup.	20
Mustard greens	1/2 cup	15
Okra	1/2 cup, cuts and pods	35
	1/2 cup, sliced	25
Onions, mature	1/2 cup	30
Parsnips	1/2 cup, diced	50
	1/2 cup, mashed	70

Calories

Peas, green	1/2 cup	65
Peppers, green	1 medium	15
Potatoes:		
Au gratin	1/2 cup	180
Baked	2 1/3-inch diameter, 4 3/4-inch	145
	long potato.	
Boiled	2 1/2-inch-diameter potato .	90
	1/2 cup, diced	55
Chips	Ten 1 3/4 x 2 1/2-inch chips .	115
French fries:		
Fresh	Ten 3 1/2 x 1/4-inch pieces .	215
Frozen	Ten 3 1/2 x 1/4-inch pieces. .	170
Hash-browned . . .	1/2 cup	175
Mashed:		
Milk added . . .	1/2 cup	70
Milk and fat added . .	1/2 cup	100
Made from granules	1/2 cup	100
with milk and		
fat added.		
Pan-fried from raw . . .	1/2 cup	230
Salad:		
Made with cooked salad	1/2 cup	125
dressing.		
Made with mayonnaise	1/2 cup	180
or		
French dressing		
and eggs.		
Scalloped without cheese .	1/2 cup	125
Sticks	1/2 cup, pieces 3/4 to 2 3/4	95
	inches long.	
Pumpkin	1/2 cup	40
Rutabagas	1/2 cup, sliced or diced . . .	30
Sauerkraut, canned . . .	1/2 cup	20
Spinach	1/2 cup	25
Squash:		
Summer	1/2 cup	15
Winter:		
Baked	1/2 cup, mashed	65
Boiled	1/2 cup, mashed	45
Sweet potatoes		
Baked in skin	5 x 2-inch potato	160
Candied	1/2 potato, 2 1/2 inches long .	160
Canned	1/2 cup, mashed	140
Tomatoes	1/2 cup	30
Tomato juice	1/2 cup	25
Tomato juice cocktail . .	1/2 cup	25
Turnips	1/2 cup, diced	20
Turnip greens	1/2 cup	15
Vegetable juice cocktail . .	1/2 cup	20
Fruits (raw):		
Apples	2 3/4-inch-diameter apple . .	80
Apricots	3 (about 1/4 pound) . . .	55
Avocados:		
California varieties . . .	Half of a 10-ounce avocado. .	190
Florida varieties	Half of a 16-ounce avocado. .	205

Calories

Bananas	One 6- to 7-inch banana (about 1/3 pound).	85
	One 8- to 9-inch banana (about 2/5 pound).	100
Berries:		
Blackberries	1/2 cup	40
Blueberries	1/2 cup	45
Raspberries, red	1/2 cup	35
Raspberries, black	1/2 cup	50
Strawberries	1/2 cup	30
Canatloup	Half of a 5-inch melon	80
Cherries:		
Sour	1/2 cup	30
Sweet	1/2 cup	40
Dates, "fresh" and dried, pitted, cut.	1/2 cup	245
Figs:		
Fresh	3 small	95
Dried	1 large	60
Grapefruit:		
White	Half of a 3 3/4-inch fruit	45
	1/2 cup sections	40
Pink or red	Half of a 3 3/4-inch fruit	50
Grapes:		
Slip skin (Concord, Delaware, Niagara, etc.).	1/2 cup	35
Adherent skin (Malaga, Thompson seedless, Flame Tokay, etc.).	1/2 cup	55
Honeydew melon	2 x 7-inch wedge	50
Oranges	2 5/8-inch orange	65
Peaches	One 2 1/2-inch peach (about 1/4 pound).	40
	1/2 cup, sliced	30
Pears	One 3 1/2 x 2 1/2-inch pear	100
Pineapple	1/2 cup, diced	40
Plums:		
Damson	Five 1-inch plums (2 ounces)	35
Japanese	One 2 1/8-inch plum (about 2 1/2 ounces).	30
Raisins	1/2 cup, packed	240
Tangerines	2 3/8-inch tangerine (about 1/4 pound).	40
Watermelon	One 2-pound wedge	110
Fruits (cooked, canned, or frozen):		
Applesauce:		
Unsweetened	1/2 cup	50
Sweetened	1/2 cup	115
Apricots:		
Canned in water	1/2 cup, halves and liquid	45
Canned in heavy syrup	1/2 cup, halves and syrup	110
Dried, cooked, unsweetened	1/2 cup, fruit and juice	105

                                                                    Calories

Berries:
    Blueberries, frozen,   1/2 cup   45
        unsweetened.
    Blueberries, frozen,   1/2 cup   120
        sweetened.
    Raspberries, red, frozen,   1/2 cup   120
        sweetened.
    Strawberries, frozen,   1/2 cup, sliced   140
        sweetened
Cherries:
    Sour, canned in water . . 1/2 cup   50
    Sweet, canned in water . . 1/2 cup   65
    Sweet, canned in syrup . . 1/2 cup   105
Figs, canned in heavy syrup . 1/2 cup   110
Fruit cocktail, canned in   1/2 cup   95
    heavy syrup.
Grapefruit, canned:
    Water pack . . . . . 1/2 cup   35
    Syrup pack . . . . . 1/2 cup   90
Peaches:
    Canned in water . . . . 1/2 cup   40
    Canned in heavy syrup . . 1/2 cup   100
    Dried, cooked, unsweetened 1/2 cup   100
    Frozen, sweetened . . . 1/2 cup   110
Pears:
    Canned in water . . . . 1/2 cup   40
    Canned in heavy syrup . . 1/2 cup   95
Pineapple, canned:
    Crushed, tidbits or chunks, 1/2 cup   95
        in heavy syrup.
    Sliced, in heavy syrup . . 2 small or 1 large slice and   80
                           2 tablespoons juice.
Plums, canned in syrup . . . 1/2 cup   105
Prunes, dried, cooked:
    Unsweetened . . . . 1/2 cup, fruit and liquid. . . 125
    Sweetened . . . . . 1/2 cup, fruit and liquid. . . 205
Rhubarb, cooked, sweetened . 1/2 cup   190
Fruit juices:
Apple juice, canned . . . . 1/2 cup   60
Grape:
    Bottled . . . . . 1/2 cup   85
    Frozen, diluted . . . 1/2 cup   65
Grapefruit:
    Fresh . . . . . . 1/2 cup   50
    Canned:
        Unsweetened . . . 1/2 cup   50
        Sweetened . . . 1/2 cup   65
    Frozen concentrate,
        ready-to-serve:
        Unsweetened . . . 1/2 cup   50
        Sweetened . . . 1/2 cup   60
Lemon, raw or canned . . . 1 tablespoon   5
Orange:
    Fresh . . . . . . 1/2 cup   55

Calories

Canned, unsweetened . .	1/2 cup	60
Frozen concentrate, ready-to-serve.	1/2 cup	55
Pineapple, canned, unsweetened	1/2 cup	70
Prune, canned	1/2 cup	100
Tangerine, canned:		
Unsweetened	1/2 cup	55
Sweetened	1/2 cup	60

IN REVIEW

1. Slimfast by selecting chewy foods which boost digestive enzyme flow and thereby metabolize more calories for better weight loss.
2. Charles O'C. lost stubborn pounds with a 5-step Slimfasting "chewy" program.
3. Chewy foods are lower in calories than refined foods.
4. Begin your Slimfasting calorie control program with a goal as to how many calories you want daily and how many pounds you want to lose. Use simple calculations as suggested.
5. Barbara Q. lost "impossible overweight" pounds on a calorie-chewing Slimfasting program.
6. The secret of "chewy" foods is the "transit time" factor.
7. Calorie planning is easy with the official U.S. Government recommendations and charts, which include portion sizes for hundreds of different foods.

Chapter Ten

How Herbs Control

Your Appetite During Slimfasting

Betty and Sophie T. insisted they were "born into a fat family" since their parents and relatives were all overweight. These two sisters were overweight as far back as they could recall. They had tried various reducing programs but both were tormented by the urge to eat. They were overweight because they could not control their appetites and so they swiftly gained back whatever was lost. They would have remained overweight, using the erroneous excuse that "fat ran in the family," except that Betty T. decided to try Slimfasting, with an emphasis on a special herb program.

HERB TONICS, HERB FLAVORINGS, HERB ELIXIRS

Betty T. prepared an assortment of herbs in the form of tonics (mixed with beverages) or for use as flavorings on smaller portions of foods, or as an elixir which combined a few simple ingredients for a tasty concoction.

HERB SLIMFASTING PROGRAM MAKES FAT "VANISH"

Betty T. followed an easy herb Slimfasting program (her scoffing sister declined) which called for these easy steps:

First Day: Cut all normal food portions in half. Begin each of the three daily meals with a *Sage Tonic* prepared by crushing 1 ounce of sage in 2 cups of boiling water. When tepid, sip 2 tablespoons. Throughout the meal, sip more of this *Sage Tonic.* At the end of the meal, use it as your beverage.

Second Day: Devote entirely to the eating of raw fresh fruits. For beverage, prepare an easy *Sassafras Elixir.* Steep the woody root bark in 2 cups of boiling water. When cool, drink slowly. Flavor with lemon juice and honey, if desired.

Third Day: Devote entirely to the eating of raw fresh vegetables. Flavor them with *parsley* (either fresh or dehydrated). Chew thoroughly. It is important to use much parsley.

Fourth Day: Devote entirely to fresh raw fruit juices that are flavored with cinnamon, peppermint, spearmint.

Fifth Day: Devote entirely to fresh raw vegetable juices that are flavored with thyme, oregano, valerian.

AT END OF HERB SLIMFASTING, OVER 18 POUNDS LOST

Just five days and Betty T. was able to lose over 18 pounds. But more important, *her appetite was under control.* Gone were gnawing hunger pangs. Forgotten were those insatiable eating urges. Eliminated were runaway appetite binges at the program's end. Betty T. now was proof to her overweight sister that "fat did NOT run in the family" but eating habits and patterns did! She had lost stubborn "inherited" weight because she had used herbs to act as "natural reducing pills" to control her appetite. Now, Betty T. uses a variety of different herbs in teas or elixirs to put a "stopgap" on her appetite. She was able to eventually shed more than 57 ugly, unwanted pounds and become slim and youthful, in contrast to her overweight sister and family. Once a month, she followed the preceding easy *Five Day Herb Slimfasting* program to help keep herself internally cleansed and in healthy balance. It is the tasty way to slim down.

HOW HERBS ARE ALL-NATURAL REDUCING PILLS

As Nature's grasses, herbs create an internal reaction so that they can control your runaway appetite and help you slim down the natural way. In effect, they act as all-natural reducing pills.

ALERTS BIOPLASM POWER OF CELLS

Herbs have the ability to stimulate and alert the bioplasm power of your body cells which influence your appetite. That is, they energize the metabolic process so that a bioplasm reaction takes place. A bioplasm reaction selects, dissolves, assimilates, metabolizes, eliminates all that enters within the cell and adipose (fat) tissues of the body. Herbs have this unique power of alerting the bioplasm reaction so that the body's own vital force can then uproot, dissolve and cast out the accumulated weighty substances in the adipose fatty tissues. This response creates an appetite satisfaction, too. It helps control the urge to eat while the cells are being slimmed down.

HIGHLY EFFECTIVE DURING SLIMFASTING

During a Slimfasting program when the metabolism has less "competition" from newly eaten foods, herbs can work without interference to create this bioplasm reducing action. Folks who are troubled by "dynamic appetite" or "stomach rumbles" will find that the use of herbs in the form of a tonic or a flavoring agent on foods will help cut down on both appetite and stomach rumbles. The bioplasm reaction of herbs will help create a comfortable feeling of fullness, even though the food intake is curtailed during Slimfasting. This helps make weight loss a delightful experience because of the "reducing pill" effect of herbs during Slimfasting.

THE HERB THAT ERASES APPETITE WHILE YOU SLIMFAST

Ned P. had a spreading paunch that gave him a "bay window" look and added years to his young appearance. He was developing an embarrassing double chin with thick, corpulent folds reaching down his chest. His basic problem was the frantic urge to eat and eat and eat. He always complained that if he could erase his appetite, he could lose the heavy paunch and age-causing jowls. He had tried a few fasting programs but he was frequently seized with the violent urge to eat. He'd grab all available food in the middle of his fasting and gulp it down. So he followed an easy Slimfasting program that called for the use of different herbs in tonics and elixirs to be taken throughout the day. This Herb Slimfasting program was aimed at striking at the *cause* of his overweight: his wild appetite.

GOLDEN SEAL HERB TONIC

Ned P. obtained golden seal herb powder. He would steep 1 ounce of the herb in 2 cups of boiled water. Lemon juice and a bit of honey would be added for flavoring. Then Ned P. would sip this Golden Seal Herb Tonic slowly, *every two hours* of the day. He discovered that his appetite almost vanished! He no longer felt the fanatical urge to eat. During his Slimfasting program, he was able to feel comfortable, satisfied and without any wild appetite.

PAUNCH FLATTENS, CHIN SLIMS DOWN, WEIGHT IS LOST

With a simple Slimfasting program calling for fresh raw fruit and vegetable juices for 17 days, Ned P. was able to see his paunch flatten, his chin firm down and his weight literally vanish from his body. He lost some 35 pounds and about 7 inches from his wasteline. Now he measured a slim 34 inches around the waist. He looked and felt years younger.

The use of the Golden Seal Herb Tonic had conquered his uncontrollable appetite.

SECRET OF HERB'S SLIMMING POWER

Ingredients in golden seal tend to soothe the mucous membranes of the mouth and the tongue. The ingredients help to tone up and sustain the venous circulation, thereby promoting better metabolism and assimilation of food. This helps create slimming. Its most effective power is upon dulling the taste buds of the tongue.

"TURNS OFF" TONGUE TASTE BUDS

The little-known secret of golden seal as an all-natural appetite-depressant is in its effect upon the taste buds of the tongue. Basically, your tongue consists of a few highly mobile muscles covered with mucous membranes that include *the taste buds*. This is the core, the foundation or the very basic root cause of your appetite. Control these taste buds and you control your appetite. Golden seal is one such herb that is able to create this natural appetite-control reaction by turning off the tongue's taste buds.

Ingredients in golden seal tend to soothe and coat the *papillae* (small, rounded elevations on the surface of the tongue) and thereby "turn off" the desire to eat. *These elevations or taste buds are thereby "coated" and "soothed" by golden seal herbal ingredients so you feel comfortably "full" and, more important, free from the urge to eat and overeat.*

Many herbs are able to soothe the urge of these papillae or tiny projections on the tongue surface and thereby act as all-natural appetite depressants. Golden seal appears to be the most effective.

HERBS: HOW TO USE THEM IN A SLIMFASTING PROGRAM

What Are Herbs? They are plant products, the leafy parts of temperate-zone plants.

How Are They Available? Individual parts are usually available. You may obtain the dried seeds, buds, fruit or flower parts, bark or roots, or a powder. Available either in these parts, or as a tea.

Where Are They Available? Most health stores will have a variety of different types of herbs. They are also available at pharmacies as well as the more specialized herbal pharmacies. Look in the classified section of your nearest large city telephone directory under such categories as "Health Stores," "Pharmacies," "Herbs," or "Herbal Pharmacies."

How Should Herbs Be Stored? In a cool, dry place in airtight containers. A warm storage area may reduce effectiveness. A damp environment creates caking, color change, and infestation. Containers should be tightly closed after each use so the volatile oils of the herb are not lost. Under favorable conditions, herbs will retain maximum aroma, flavor, and reducing-ability up to six months. Whole herbs keep their potency much longer.

How Should Herbs Be Used? Generally speaking, about 1/8 teaspoon per pint of boiled water for a tea. If adding to food, plan for 1/4 teaspoon per pound of the main item or a pint of sauce.

How Can Herbs Be Used for Slimfasting? Select any of the herbs listed in this chapter. Use 1/8 of a teaspoon per pint of boiling water. Use lemon juice and honey for taste. Drink several pints of this herbal tea throught the day as a means of easing your appetite urge and making you feel "comfortable" and "full" even on a lowered food intake.

Herbs are able to control your appetite and keep you alert and vigorous while pounds melt away from your body. They are considered "all-natural reducing pills."

FOUR BASIC TYPES OF SLIMFASTING HERBS

Depending upon your tastes and needs, select any of these types of Slimfasting herbs that are available at most herbal outlets:

1. *Roots and Barks.* Simmer roots for 30 or more minutes in order to extract their Slimfasting values. Do not boil hard. NOTE: If you gather the roots and barks yourself, cut or crush them fine. If you raise or gather herbs and barks, use good judgment in making teas. If you get it too strong, add more freshly boiled water.

2. *Flowers and Leaves.* Do not boil. Steep flowers and leaves in boiling water in a covered dish for 20 minutes, just as you would brew ordinary tea. Boiling evaporates the aromatic and Slimfasting properties.

3. *Powdered Herbs.* Mix in freshly boiled water or in fruit or vegetable juice. The Slimfasting effect is more pronounced if taken in boiled water. Drink only when comfortably tepid.

4. *Capsule, Tablet.* Most health stores and pharmacies have herbs available as a capsule or tablet. Take several per day (see directions on container) during your Slimfasting program.

Suggestions: Powdered herbs may be mixed with foods such as mashed potatoes or mashed vegetables of any kind, sweet fruits such as figs or dates, or mashed together with them. You may always use a little honey for added flavor with herbs. *Never* use refined or any other kind of sugar for flavoring or for any other reason!

How Herbs Create Slimfasting Weight Loss

During the growth process, the roots of the herb literally suck up nourishment from the soil. The roots have many small mouths that "eat and drink" the important nutrients from the soil.

In the form of fluid, this liquid or "sap" then goes up into the stalk of the herb where it nourishes the plant. Everything in the herb plant, including its bark, wood, leaves, flowers, and fruit, is made from this sap that travels upward to serve as nourishment.

This sap is considered Nature's perfect food! It sustains the plant which needs almost no other nourishment except for water and sunshine. It keeps the plant alive. It is this same sap that is found in the herb which you consume. It helps stabilize your body processes. It organizes your hormonal responses. It helps control overeating. Just as an herbal plant rejects excess food, so will your body reject excess food during Slimfasting if it is adequately fortified with herbs.

HERB PLANT IS LIVING FACTORY

Compare the herb plant to your body and see how the "sap" can be used to create the same health within your system as within the plant. The sap goes up one route to the leaves, then down to the roots through another route. Compare it to the way your blood (sap) travels along the route (arteries) from your heart and then back to your heart through the veins (route). Therefore, herb "sap" is comparable to human sap or blood.

Herbal sap nourishes the plant, keeping it healthy and alive.

Human sap (blood) nourishes your entire body, every part of your organism.

When you introduce herbal sap (plant blood) into your system, you restore a natural balance that helps stabilize your metabolic-assimilative processes and Slimfasting is then able to take place.

A GARDEN OF SLIMFASTING HERBS

Select any of these and use them throughout your Slimfasting program. They will help control your appetite, ease hunger urge, and set off a chain reaction that will melt away pounds and shrink down inches.

ALOES

How to Use: Use in the form of a tonic with freshly boiled water or add to a fresh fruit or vegetable juice. Use in the morning to help control appetite at the start of the day.

Slimfasting Benefits: A fine body cleanser; helps scrub away weighty matter from many of the body organs. Helps loosen and cast out weight from the body through eliminative channels.

ANGELICA

How to Use: Delightful in the form of a tea, either from the roots or the seeds. Steep for 20 minutes. Flavor with lemon juice and honey.

Slimfasting Benefits: Ingredients tend to soothe stomach rumbles, create a feeling of comfortable fullness and natural appetite control.

ANISE

How to Use: Mix with or take with other herbs as a tonic.

Slimfasting Benefits: Helps guard against fermentation of accumulated wastes in the digestive system; eases stomach grumbles so there is little "empty stomach syndrome" during weight loss.

BALM

How to Use: As a tea with flavoring. This is the most effective method.

Slimfasting Benefits: Ingredients in balm (also available as sweet balm, lemon balm, garden balm) tend to induce perspiration. This is most important since body pores need to be opened so weighty materials loosened can be cast out and slimming occur.

BASIL, SWEET

How to Use: Sprinkle in beverages or use as a tea.

Slimfasting Benefits: Through its vitamin action, helps to trigger a stepped-up glandular reaction so that fat-melting hormones can help burn up accumulated weight.

BAYBERRY

How to Use: Either bark, leaves or flowers can be used as a tea or sprinkled over fruit or vegetable salads.

Slimfasting Benefits: Herbal ingredients tend to increase forms of mucous secretions that coat the tongue's papillae and thereby nullify the urge to want to eat. By shielding these taste buds and temporarily putting them "to sleep," bayberry is able to act as a natural appetite suppressant.

BAY LEAVES

How to Use: Steep in boiled water for a tonic. Use as a flavoring for cooked foods. Just halve food portions. You'll feel satisfaction because of aromatic properties in bay leaves even with lesser amounts.

Slimfasting Benefits: Herbal "sap" tends to cleanse the system and acts as an astringent for the adipose cell tissues to promote weight loss.

BEECH

How to Use: As a tonic in boiled water or in fruit or vegetable juice.

Slimfasting Benefits: Tones up the entire system but has an important bioplasm power whereby cells are scrubbed and reduced to promote weight loss.

BITTER ROOT

How to Use: Tasty in the form of an elixir in boiled water with some lemon juice and honey.

Slimfasting Benefits: Ingredients create water loss: this acts as a natural diuretic so sodium-carrying water can be cast out of the body and help create slimming.

BLUE FLAG

How to Use: Sprinkle over fruits and vegetables.

Slimfasting Benefits: Creates a feeling of "appetite euphoria" so that during fasting there is a feeling of quietude and relaxation. Helps act as a natural appetite depressant.

BORAGE

How to Use: Take as a tea with lemon juice and honey.

Slimfasting Benefits: Ingredients tend to cleanse the blood and also expel toxic wastes that are removed from adipose tissues during the fasting program.

BURDOCK

How to Use: Either as a tea or sprinkle into fruit or vegetable juices. Also sprinkle the crushed root over raw fruit salad.

Slimfasting Benefits: Properties in the root tend to act as a diuretic to wash out accumulated sediment from the system. This helps remove weighty substances and bring down pounds and shrink inches from many body parts.

CAMOMILE

How to Use: A fragrant tonic with honey and lemon juice.

Slimfasting Benefits: Soothes and heals the broken or damaged body cells. Also helps to create internal regularity and a feeling of comfort so that there is no unnatural desire for food.

CARAWAY

How to Use: Add as a flavoring to baked and other foods. Good in steamed brown rice or in a pudding with brown rice. Helpful during a Slimfasting program of brown rice and fruit.

Slimfasting Benefits: Protects against fermentation of accumulated wastes in the digestive system and promotes better enzymatic digestion of ingested fats, calories and carbohydrates. Helps cast out debris and waste.

CASCARA

How to Use: In moderation as a pungent tonic.

Slimfasting Benefits: Ingredients create a strong and powerful expelling action upon the intestinal region. Helps establish regularity and rids the body of accumulated wastes; this creates a healthy "shrinkage" of pounds and inches. Also tends to "fill up" the digestive tract and give a feeling of comfortable fullness.

CELERY

How to Use: Try the root and the seed as a flavoring for soups or for a hot broth.

Slimfasting Benefits: Creates a form of natural perspiration, so that this diuretic action will wash out accumulated debris. Helps soothe the nervous system so there is a markedly reduced desire for eating.

COLTSFOOT

How to Use: Boil roots and leaves and use as a vegetable.

Slimfasting Benefits: Creates a natural appetite control reaction by soothing the organs involved in digestion. Tends to "swell" so there is a simultaneous reaction of fullness.

COMFREY

How to Use: Use the root or leaves for a tea.

Slimfasting Benefits: Herb contains *allantoin. Allantoin* will scrub the cells and then help them repair themselves in the adipose tissue rejuvenation process. Therefore, it slims you down while helping to make you look and feel youthful.

CORIANDER

How to Use: Seeds make a tasty tea; may also be used as a broth.

Slimfasting Benefits: Acts as a good digestive tonic to ease rumbles so that there is a contented feeling during a reducing program.

DANDELION

How to Use: Leaves and roots may be used for a salad; or boil as part of a broth.

Slimfasting Benefits: Ingredients tend to purify the bloodstream and control acid-alkaline levels in the system. The root helps the body create water loss (natural diuretic) so the weighty substances are washed out through eliminative channels.

FENNEL

How to Use: Flavor salads and also sprinkle over other foods. Steep in boiled water and take as a tonic.

Slimfasting Benefits: Herbal ingredients tend to relieve spasms and so-called cramps and increase water dispersion of the system. Helps allay hunger while serving to cleanse the body of weighty wastes.

FENUGREEK

How to Use: Seeds make a tasty tea. The boiled seeds may be used in a salad; they offer good nourishment.

Slimfasting Benefits: Has a mucilaginous reaction; that is, coats the system with a soothing substance so that there is a protective covering against irritants. At the same time, the expanded seeds tend to "fill up" to create appetite satisfaction so there is less hunger.

FLAXSEED

How to Use: Seeds can be steeped for a tea; also use boiled seeds as part of a raw salad.

Slimfasting Benefits: Create a demulcent (soothing) reaction upon digestive organs so there is a markedly reduced appetite-hunger urge.

GENTIAN ROOT

How to Use: Use the dried root in the form of a powder for a tonic.

Slimfasting Benefits: Offers a mucilaginous reaction so there is a soothing response and digestive organs feel contented. Helps cleanse out toxic wastes from the system.

GINGER

How to Use: Chew the root to stimulate salivary glands, to coat the papillae of the tongue, and to help soothe the urge to overeat.

Slimfasting Benefits: When taken hot, in a tea or broth, creates a diaphoretic (perspiration) response. This helps the body cleanse itself of accumulated water, which slims down adipose tissues.

GINSENG

How to Use: Chew the fresh root, or take in the form of a tea.

Slimfasting Benefits: Acts as a natural tranquilizer for the digestive organs so there is a markedly reduced appetite. Also appears to regulate glandular-hormonal secretions for better metabolism.

GOLDEN SEAL

How to Use: Prepare a tea from the powder, combine with mint for good flavor.

Slimfasting Benefits: Exerts a special influence on the mucous membranes and tissues, thereby coating the organs and easing the urge for excess food.

HOREHOUND

How to Use: As a tea, or as a syrup which is prepared by boiling the leaves and roots in a smaller amount of water.

Slimfasting Benefits: Acts by soothing the desire to overeat, coats the papillae of the tongue and also the oral tissues which often have a tendency to promote nervous eating.

JUNIPER BERRIES

How to Use: Boil bark for tea. Use boiled berries as a fruit or as a topping for raw salads.

Slimfasting Benefits: Creates a natural diuretic action; helps alert a self-scrubbing of the cells to promote reduction.

MAGNOLIA

How to Use: Boil bark for tea.

Slimfasting Benefits: Creates a febrifuge response, which creates an antipyretic or inflammation-soothing benefit for the fasting person.

MARJORAM

How to Use: A flavorful tea.

Slimfasting Benefits: Very effective when combined with camomile and gentian as a tea; this combination tends to increase water loss from the body and thereby cleanse the system and scrub cells and tissues for healthy rejuvenation during weight loss.

MINT

How to Use: Crush the leaves and sprinkle over raw fruit or vegetable salads; also use for a tea.

Slimfasting Benefits: Exerts a refreshing "taste" that soothes the buds of the tongue. This acts as a natural self-control over the eating urge.

MULLEIN

How to Use: Make a tea from the leaves.

Slimfasting Benefits: Very soothing to the circulatory-respiratory systems so that there is a marked reduction in the urge to overeat. Helps control appetite.

PARSLEY

How to Use: Either use the powder for a tea or eat the leaves and crushed root with a raw salad.

Slimfasting Benefits: Creates a natural febrifuge response. During fasting, there may be a feverish-inflamed feeling which is soothed-cooled by parsley.

PEPPERMINT

How to Use: Leaves make a tasty tea. Also use peppermint oil as a body rub to cleanse the skin pores.

Slimfasting Benefits: Acts as a natural stimulant; that is, ingredients act powerfully within the system, diffusing throughout the circulatory system so that metabolism is alerted. Furthermore, the pleasant peppermint taste helps soothe the taste buds of the mouth and control the appetite.

RED CLOVER

How to Use: Infuse as a tea. Combine with a bit of apple cider vinegar.

Slimfasting Benefits: Acts as an oral astringent so that the mouth and throat feel cleansed of debris. This also soothes the mucous membranes and eases the desire to overeat.

ROSEMARY

How to Use: Crush the leaves for use as a tea.

Slimfasting Benefits: Helps soothe and ease stomach spasms and rumbles so there are less of the annoying "hunger cramps" than with most slimming programs. Gentle to the system and exerts a tranquil feeling.

SAGE

How to Use: Excellent as a tea.

Slimfasting Benefits: Appears to control circulatory secretions and helps to quiet and soothe the digestive system. Offers relaxation of the muscles that might otherwise churn up in the desire for food.

SARSAPARILLA

How to Use: Use as a tea, or use powdered root to sprinkle over raw salads.

Slimfasting Benefits: Acts as a natural sedative in soothing the appetite: appears to influence the glands so there is more internal harmony and better emotional control over the compulsive eating urge.

SASSAFRAS

How to Use: Use the bark of the root for a tea infusion; also crush and sprinkle over salads.

Slimfasting Benefits: Appears to purify the blood and cleanse the other systems and helps to calm down internal spasms and so-called hunger eruptions.

SENNA

How to Use: Delicious as a tea, also sprinkle crumpled leaves over raw salads.

Slimfasting Benefits: Acts as a mild expellant of accumulated wastes and thereby cleanses the system. Cleanses the cells and tissues, performing a scrubbing reaction. Also soothes appetite buds.

SPEARMINT

How to Use: Any part of the plant may be used for brewing tea, chewing, or sprinkling over raw salads.

Slimfasting Benefits: Refreshes the mouth and tongue so there is a healthy feeling of appetite satisfaction.

THYME

How to Use: The leaves may be crushed for tea or used on a salad.

Slimfasting Benefits: Helps induce perspiration so that wastes are removed. Also appears to create an emotional tranquility so there is a marked appetite reduction.

YARROW

How to Use: Helpful if taken in the morning as a tea.

Slimfasting Benefits: Creates a natural diuretic response. Helps soothe the nervous system if taken early in the day and puts a natural "stopgap" on the appetite.

Herbs have soil-nourished ingredients that act as a natural appetite-depressant. Whether taken in the form of tonics or flavorings, they are effective in helping to control your appetite as well as erase hunger sensations during your Slimfasting program.

IN REVIEW

1. Fat sisters, Betty and Sophie T., discovered that fat does *not* "run in the family." Betty T. lost more than 57 unwanted pounds on a Five Day Herb Slimfasting program while her doubting sister remained overweight.

2. Herbs exert the bioplasm reaction by promoting birth and rebirth of cellular matter, thereby regenerating from within. Herbs ease appetite and control hunger urges during Slimfasting.

3. Ned P. lost some 35 pounds and 7 inches on an herb Slimfasting program.

4. Golden Seal Herb Tonic is able to "turn off" tongue taste buds and control appetite on any Slimfasting program.

5. It's easy to obtain and use herbs as described in this chapter.

6. Select any of the four basic types of Slimfasting herbs for your own use.

7. Enjoy any herbs from the "garden" listing. All are easy to use. All offer you Slimfasting benefits.

Chapter Eleven

How to Use Behavior Therapy ("BT") to Stay Slim Forever and Ever

Behavior therapy (BT) is a method that calls for retraining of certain habits to help overcome obstacles and barriers that inhibit success. The overweight person will often need to resort to the use of behavior therapy or "BT" because of backsliding in a slimming program or inability to stick to Slimfasting until results are achieved.

CHANGE YOUR BEHAVIOR PATTERN

Part of the behavioral approach to weight loss under Slimfasting involves an understanding of what you eat, when and where you eat it, and how much. Under Slimfasting, you may be eating all the raw fruits you wish and you still feel hungry and have an insatiable urge to eat other foods. By changing your behavior pattern, you can re-educate your "situation control" and feel no unnatural hunger as you Slimfast. The important thing is *not* in the eating of the foods on your Slimfasting program. Instead, the *method* of eating is the key to satisfaction and contentment and eventual weight loss. Change your behavior pattern and you can stay slim forever and ever!

TWO BASIC "BT" TECHNIQUES TO CREATE FAST WEIGHT LOSS

Eva Mc. had gone on an easy 5-day Slimfasting program that called for alternating days of raw fruit and vegetable juices. These were flavored with herbs as seasonings. Eva Mc. also used herbal tonics, yet she found that she still had that compulsive urge to eat and overeat. Eva Mc. kept gaining back lost pounds and inches. She needed a simple behavior therapy or "BT" adjustment that would make Slimfasting a successful weight losing program without any hunger urge. She followed these two basic "BT" techniques:

1. *Where to Eat.* During any Slimfasting program, eat ONLY

in a proper eating place. This may be at the kitchen table, at the dining room table, or at any other table. But you must eat *only* in this place. *Benefit:* This eliminates the compulsive eater's urge to taste food as it is cooking on the stove. It also eliminates the urge to snack or nibble while watching television or lying in bed.

2.   *How to Eat.* During any Slimfasting program, follow an *unhurried eating style.* Even if you are on a juice fast, do this casually and leisurely. Be aware of each mouthful from the minute it leaves your plate or glass until it is finally swallowed. This means reversing a lifetime of rushing through meals. *Benefit:* When you chew, chew and swallow (juices should be savored in your mouth before you swallow), you eliminate the gulp-and-swallow pattern that is often the cause of overweight. An unhurried style offers you a great deal of satisfaction and soothes the urge to want to overeat. Eat each bite of food, slowly chewing thoroughly before swallowing. Rest between bites. During the time of eating, savor and think about the taste of the food. This gives you much emotional and physical satisfaction. On any Slimfasting program, you will find yourself "filled up" with these two basic techniques.

APPETITE SATISFIED, POUNDS MELT, INCHES SHRINK

Eva Mc. used these two basic behavior therapy or "BT" techniques during her Slimfasting program and discovered that she felt almost no unnatural hunger. There was no agonizing urge to overeat. After five days, she weighed herself. Many pounds had actually "melted" from her body. She tape-measured herself. Unsightly inches had "shrunk" and she now had a healthy and youthful figure. Thanks to these two basic "BT" techniques, she had used mind-body influences to help her become slim and stay slim forever and ever under regular Slimfasting.

Weigh Yourself Daily: Set Your Goals

If you find that under Slimfasting that you still lack strong emotional control, you may use simple behavior therapy programs to help protect you from being a "diet dropout." To begin with, it is important that you weigh yourself daily to see how much you have (or have not) lost. Then you set your goals. Here's how:

Slimfast regularly, with a minimum of seven days per month. Your goal is to reach your desired or ideal weight level. When you have reached that level, you slowly return to eating formerly forbidden or taboo foods. Enjoy chocolate eclairs and ice cream sodas, if you prefer. *Under Slimfasting, you can indulge in favorite cakes and pies provided you do not eat more calories than you burn and do not gain back lost weight.* That is why you need to Slimfast regularly and also *weigh yourself daily* to guard against creeping overweight.

IF YOUR SCALES SHOW WEIGHT GAIN:

Immediately go on a Slimfasting program with *reduced* amounts of foods so that you can lose this added weight.

This gives you a balance. You will not actually be counting calories. Instead, your body will *show* calories in the form of this added weight. *Under no circumstances should you let yourself gain more than four unwanted or unnecessary pounds.* By checking your weight daily, you will be using simple behavior therapy that helps make reducing an easy accomplishment.

SEVEN STEP BEHAVIOR THERAPY SLIMFASTING PROGRAM FOR FAST "FOREVER SLIM" WEIGHT LOSS

Charles Y. had successfully lost weight under a raw vegetable Slimfasting program. He found that with daily weighing, he kept gaining back more and more pounds after his slimming session. He needed to readjust his methods of eating. So it was that Charles Y. used "BT" or behavior therapy that not only helped him lose his 49 unwanted pounds and some eight inches from his chest, hips, and thighs, but he was "forever slim" under the program.

Here is the *7-Step Behavior Therapy Slimfasting Program* that helped Charles Y. feel "filled up" with "appetite satisfaction" as the weight and inches literally vanished from his body—for good:

Before You Begin: It is important to re-train your behavior by breaking your patterns down into very small but manageable segments. Go through them step by step. Compare it to the act of learning how to drive. You must constantly monitor your eating. This alerts you to your Slimfasting and subconsciously makes you aware of your goals toward weight loss.

1. *Write Everything Down.* In a notebook, write *everything* down. This includes all the foods you eat, all the beverages you drink. Write down the items as well as the quantities. Do this within 20 minutes after you eat, every time that you eat. Each night, look over this list to see what you did wrong, such as overeating or indulging in high-calorie foods in large quantities. When you can *see* what you have eaten, your thought patterns will change and you will then learn to avoid erroneous eating the next day.

2. *Stick to Your Slimfasting Schedule.* When you have outlined your Slimfasting program, whether for 2, 4 or 7 days or more, decide you will stick to it with NO alterations. Write down the Slimfasting schedule. Prepare it in the form of an airplane timetable. List everything, hour by hour. Break it down to specifics such as: Fruit Juice at 7:30 a.m. Herbal Tonic at 9 a.m. Fruit Salad at noon, and so forth. Decide at the outset that you will stick to this timetable just as an airplane would do. No changes. It becomes easier and more successful if you have it written down like a schedule.

3. *Be Wise When Shopping and Storing Food.* The secret to successful weight loss is NOT to have any high-calorie or forbidden foods in the house at all! This begins by being wise when you go shopping. Prepare a list in advance. DO NOT include junk food. Decide that you will NOT buy anything that is not on your shopping list. Do your shopping speedily, efficiently. Do not "eye shop" among forbidden foods. Avoid those counters or shelves. Buy what you need and leave the market. At home, try to avoid having any food before your eyes. This tempts you to eat. Store food in brown paper bags, aluminum foil, non-transparent containers. If you cannot see the food, you cannot be tempted to snack or nibble or overeat.

4. *Reschedule Your Methods of Eating.* The basics of "BT" call for adjusting your "situation control" method of eating. You'll avoid temptation and also be *rewarded with satisfaction* if you follow these BT suggestions:

- *Sit Down When Eating.* You should NOT "eat on the run." You should NOT stand, walk, or ride when eating. Instead, whenever you eat or drink on any Slimfasting program, you MUST sit down. This makes you more aware of your food intake. This creates greater appetite-stomach satisfaction.

- *Prepare a Comfortable Table Setting.* Even if you drink one glass of a beverage, do so at a table with a plate, a spoon, an attractive napkin. This gives you visual satisfaction and comfort. An attractive table setting can make the simplest food or beverage feel like a sumptuous feast.

- *Avoid Any Distractions.* When you eat or drink, do nothing else. No work. No television. No reading. No radio. No talking, except to a table partner in comfortable conversations.

- *Begin With a Glass of Water.* This helps ease the customary urge to gulp down food. It also activates your satiety mechanism so you are satisfied on Slimfasting foods and/or drinks. A glass of water before you eat will take the sharp edge off your hunger.

5. *Slower Eating Creates Better Weight Loss.* Under Slimfasting, your digestive-satiety mechanisms function better with slower eating; the fat-melting process is increased during slower eating. A simple Behavior Therapy method calls for putting your spoon or fork *down on the plate* after each swallow. Pick it up again when your mouth is empty and you're ready to eat. If you eat with your hands, put down the item (fruit or vegetable or other food) after each mouthful. If you are drinking, put down the glass after every swallow. *Benefits:* Slow-motion eating enables your digestive system to secrete more enzymes needed for fat mobilization and dispersion; also, slow-motion eating creates an emotional reaction wherein you will feel "full" even with smaller portions.

6. *Leave Some Portions on Your Plate.* Much overweight stems from an early childhood order to "finish everything" or "join the clean plate club." Reverse this situation by letting some uneaten portion remain on your plate. This is especially helpful if your eyes are still bigger than your stomach and you select a lot of food and then feel you must eat it all up. Not so! Re-train your attitudes. Select smaller portions. Then leave something on your plate. The more left over, the more successful you will be in cutting down portions. DO NOT give anyone (not even the family pet) your leftovers! Let them go to costly waste in the garbage. Reason? Leftover food means wasted money. This also means that next time you'll prepare and eat less food to avoid this waste!

7. *Adjust Your Habits.* During any Slimfasting program, your behavioral attitudes should be adjusted to accelerate weight-inches loss. Here are some suggestions:

- *Low-Calorie Fruits for Dessert.* After one or two days of Slimfasting, your taste buds will have less craving for sugary desserts. Switch to low-calorie fruits that are naturally sweet and low in calories.

- *Limit Yourself to One Helping Only.* If you feel compelled to take a "second helping," then re-train yourself this way: Divide a small portion into halves. Eat one portion, then eat the other portion as your "second helping."

- *Use Small Plates.* Behaviorally speaking, *eye appeal* can do much to either increase or decrease your appetite. Put your Slimfasting food on a very small salad plate; let it overflow. Visually, it will look like a great deal. When you finish, this perceptual trick will make smaller amounts of food seem as satisfying as if they were much larger.

By readjusting your attitudes, recognizing lifelong patterns, using BT or behavior therapy, you can help your body lose unwanted pounds and inches. It is the natural way for fast "forever slim" weight loss.

HOW TO SOLVE EMOTIONAL
EATING PROBLEMS WITH BEHAVIOR THERAPY

During some Slimfasting programs, you may have emotional disturbances that make you feel edgy or nervous or "going off the deep end." Here are some dieting problems and their behavior therapy solutions through Slimfasting:

Behavior Problem: You may feel *hunger pangs* or gnawing appetite during a slimming program.

Slimfasting Solution: Select a Slimfasting program that calls for three separate meals, even if they consist of beverages alone. Make each meal a special event. You can retrain your body and your mind so it will feel as if you are having a satisfying meal.

Behavior Problem: If you are reducing by yourself, you may feel very *lonely* or deprived or isolated.

Slimfasting Solution: A simple BT remedy is to have a long list of close friends available; call them throughout the day. Visit neighbors. Chat over the back fence. Participate in social activities. Mix with as many people as possible to get your mind off your dieting and onto others.

Behavior Problem: There are times when you feel below par, either *bored* or downright *depressed* during a reducing program.

Slimfasting Solution: Take an interest in hobbies, clubs, charities. Have a few hobbies. Plunge into books and magazines. Occupy your mind. Keed your body active through housework or other chores.

Behavior Problem: Because of the change in eating, you may feel temperamental, *angry,* on edge.

Slimfasting Solution: Tell yourself repeatedly in advance that you will be sensitive and then gird your loins (mental and physical) for tense situations. Try to avoid people and circumstances that may irritate you. Do some physical work to give vent to any feelings of anger.

Behavior Problem: There are times when you will feel worn and *fatigued.*

Slimfasting Solution: Plan ahead to have a minimum of eight (or more, if needed) hours of sleep every night. This is your iron-clad rule. No cheating! This will give you needed rest. You may want to take occasional naps during the day.

Learn to *recognize the cause* of your behavioral problem and then plan to *correct the cause* so you can cope safely, easily, and happily throughout weight-losing Slimfasting.

HOW TO USE "THOUGHT CONTROL" FOR WEIGHT CONTROL

Julie O'B. used a 6-day Slimfasting program during which she would begin with raw juice fasting, then raw fruit and vegetables, then slightly cooked vegetables, and gradually ease into more solid foods such as grains, some fish, dairy products, poultry, meats. If she followed this easy once-a-month 6-day Slimfasting program, she could keep herself at a slim 120 pounds. But her problem was that she kept "visualizing" large amounts of heavy, fattening foods. No sooner did she end her program than she would rush into overeating and gain back more than 30 pounds. It was a see-saw or "yo-yo" problem. Julie O'B. needed to use thought control for weight control. She followed a "respondent treatment" which used BT or behavior therapy that controlled and eventually eliminated the visions of so-called forbidden foods. Here is this same method of thought control that can re-adjust your thinking patterns so that you'll be "turned off" at the prospect of overeating.

Respondent Treatment for "Thought Control"

What Is It? A method that pairs one positive thought with one negative thought.

How Does It Control Appetite? When you pair two stimuli of *unlike* values, you create a negative stimulus. Therefore, when you visualize gobs of forbidden sweet or fatty foods, you then visualize becoming violently sick after eating them. Using thought control you can actually frighten yourself away from eating the forbidden foods under threat of being sick.

What Is a Simple Example? As a youngster you probably assumed that eating chocolate would give you pimples on your face. Therefore, you passed up eating chocolates so that you would not have the social stigma of a pimply face. Follow this same analogy in reducing. Visualize the negative consequences of eating taboo foods and you'll be turned off.

How Can "Thought Control" Be Used During Slimfasting? If you find yourself visually excited over foods either before, during, or after Slimfasting, try some of these do-it-yourself thought control behavior therapy programs:

Bad Odor Aversive Stimulus. Carry along a vial of some substance that has a bad odor. (Nothing toxic or chemical, please!) Your pharmacist may be able to prepare it for you. Whenever you have thoughts of gooey, sweet, or fatty foods, take out the vial and breathe in the bad odor.

Covert Sensitization Technique. Whenever you imagine a problematic food, immediately change your thoughts to something very unpleasant. Think of nausea. Think of a serious and disastrous accident. Think of a tragedy. Or else think of infidelity by your mate!

Breath Holding Aversive Method. As soon as a taboo food enters your thoughts, quickly hold your breath for as long as you can! This will divert your thoughts and condition you to dislike the taboo food.

Pins and Needles Punishment. Carry a set of pins, needles, thumbtacks (or some sandpaper) with you. If you feel a food thought taking hold, reach into this bag and scratch yourself. Just a slight needle-sharp touch should "shock" you out of the desire. It is a form of punishment for being "wicked" and thinking about food. It is a simplified type of electroshock aversion used in laboratories for heavy overweight.

Retrain and re-educate your thoughts. Use these simple, but effective behavior therapy programs during Slimfasting and you will be able to insulate and shield yourself from the urge to overeat.

Use this respondent treatment by pairing one good thought with one unpleasant thought. Or, putting it simply, visualize *punishment* for partaking of any forbidden food!

The use of behavior therapy is a special adjunct to planned weight loss. It helps connect mind and body. Together, both can help you stay slim forever and ever with Slimfasting!

SUMMARY

1. Change your behavior pattern so that Slimfasting can help you lose weight fast and without emotional upset.

2. Eva Mc. used two basic "BT" or behavior therapy techniques to create fast weight loss.

3. Weigh yourself daily: Set your goals. If your scales show weight gain, go on a Slimfasting program with reduced amounts until you go back to desired level.

4. Charles Y. lost stubborn pounds on an easy 7-step behavior therapy program. It gave him a "filled up" response with "appetite satisfaction." Weight and inches vanished permanently.

5. Check your own emotional behavior problem and then the suggested Slimfasting solution.

6. Julie O'B. keeps at a permanent slim 120 pounds with a 6-day Slimfasting program that also uses "thought control."

7. Use the respondent treatment to help erase visions and obsessions of forbidden foods.

Chapter Twelve

How a Salt-Free Slimfasting Program
Creates Swift Weight Loss

Overweight pounds will actually "wash out" of your body when you follow a simple but highly effective salt-free Slimfasting program. For many overweights, salt may be more of the cause than sugar. After checking with your doctor on your salt problem, you can bring down the accumulated salt levels with reduction of this seasoning in foods, either prepared by you or processed. In so doing, your metabolism can then help "evaporate" the accumulated salt in your adipose cells and thereby "wash out" overweight from your body.

SALT: CELL-FATTENING CAUSE OF OVERWEIGHT

Most of the salt taken into your body is from the shaker or added to foods as a flavoring substance or preservative. When salt enters your system, it is transported to your intestinal tract where it remains at a storage site until the bloodstream removes it to be sent to other parts of your body.

Salt retained by your body is added to your blood plasma or to your *interstitial fluid* (the fluid which lies outside the billions of body cells). Here, the salt actually becomes absorbed in your adipose cell tissues, making them fat. *The more salt that is absorbed by these cells, the more they expand in size and the more you put on weight.* A high-salt diet means that your adipose cell tissues will become engorged and swollen and that your scale shows you are putting on more and more weight. Salt, therefore, may be as much (if not more) a cause of overweight as sugar.

SALT-FREE SLIMFASTING SLIMS DOWN CELLS

When you follow a simple salt-free Slimfasting program, your metabolism is then able to alert your *extracellular fluid* (the fluid which lies between the cells) to create a "washing" action. That is, the extracellular fluid is able to wash away the excess of salt from your billions of cells, and then actually excrete this salt through your eliminative channels. This helps to create a cell-slimming action that will bring about weight loss.

Slimfasting Reaction: When salt is restricted from your eating plan, the reserves within the cells are now being drawn upon. The fasting organism will utilize much of the stored up salt. A salt-free Slimfasting program enables your body to take out the reserves of salt, transport them through the bloodstream, and cast them out of the body. Your extracellular fluid is then able to wash your cells and drain out more excess salt. This creates a simultaneous cell-slimming and body-slimming reward.

KIDNEYS EXCRETE WEIGHT-CAUSING SALT

Your kidneys will then excrete excessive amounts of weight-causing salt. It is important for you to drink lots of fresh fruit and vegetable juices and other healthy beverages on a salt-free Slimfasting program to help your kidneys wash away the accumulated brine from your system.

Salt creates a hydraulic effect by retaining more fluid in and around and outside the cells and this creates overweight, among other body disturbances.

During Slimfasting, the reduction of salt intake will reduce this hydraulic effect, will reduce the absorption in the cells and thereby stimulate swift and permanent weight loss.

A Simple Salt-Free Slimfasting Program
Melts Lifelong Pounds, Inches

As far back as Bertha L. could remember, she had always been overweight. Now, as she approached her middle years, she decided to do something about her corpulence. She was ashamed of her "elephant thighs" as some neighbors giggled behind her back. She almost wept as she saw the scale going higher and higher. At 202 pounds, she had unsightly pounds, bulges, and inches. She had to wear long-sleeved dresses and very long skirts to hide the spreading inches all over her upper arms, her thighs and even her legs. When her chin sagged, Bertha L. was faced with a choice: continue gaining weight and become an ashamed hermit hiding indoors or behind much clothing, or go on a reducing program that would get rid of these lifelong pounds and inches.

SIMPLE ADJUSTMENT TURNS THE OVERWEIGHT TIDE

Bertha L. heard that if she could reduce the amount of stored up salt in her cells, she could simultaneously reduce weight and lose unwanted, age-causing pounds and inches. She went on a very simple Slimfasting program: *reduce or eliminate all foods containing added salt*. Bertha L. could eat most of her favorite foods, including lean meats, poultry, dairy products, even breads and pastries (provided they were salt-free; in the case of pastries, they were either very low-calorie or sugar-free), but had to eliminate intake of foods prepared with salt or with a high salt content. It was the most delicious Slimfasting reducing program Bertha L. had ever tried.

SALT LOSS = WEIGHT LOSS

During this simple salt-free Slimfasting program, the extracellular fluid was able to wash away the accumulated salt in the billions of body cells that had made Bertha L. so unsightly corpulent. Because there was a "salt fasting" program, the extracellular fluid was basically salt-free. Therefore, when it washed the adipose cell tissues, it did so with clean fluids that did not deposit salt but, instead, absorbed that which was in the cells and then helped wash it out through the kidneys and the eliminative channels. As salt was removed, Bertha L. could actually see pounds wash right out of her system. Inches began to shrink. Her waistline trimmed down. Slowly, the heavy-hanging fat began to "melt" away from her upper arms, her bust, her waistline, her thighs, her legs. Much sooner than she expected, she had actually lost over 50 pounds and many, many inches! Most joyful of all was being able to eat many of her favorite foods with just the "salt-free" restriction.

WEIGHT DROPS, INCHES VANISH

Bertha L. continued on her salt-free Slimfasting program for over 30 days. Soon, the scales showed she was a trim 122. Her waistline was a neat 32. Inches actually *vanished* from her arms, legs and other body parts. She could soon wear a size 14 dress—and it was too large, in a short time, as more weight went out of her body! Now Bertha L. is able to keep slim and trim, and she boasts of having won the battle of the bulge on her easy salt-free Slimfasting program. It's a delicious way to remain permanently slim.

HOW TO PLAN YOUR SALT-FREE
SLIMFASTING PROGRAM

The less salt your cells absorb, the less weight you will gain. Begin by selecting foods that are basically low in salt or sodium. Note the counts in Figure 12-1.

PRACTICE SCORECARD

RESTRICTIONS

	Item	Size of Serving	Other ( )	Calories	Mgs. Sodium
BREAKFAST	corn flakes—low-salt	1 cup		90	10
	skim milk	8 ozs.		80	100
	cantaloupe	1/4 melon		30	12
	orange juice	8 ozs.		100	3
LUNCH	flounder or sole	3 1/2 ozs.		68	56
	brown rice	1/4 cup		160	3
	apple	1 medium		80	1
	grapes	22		69	3
	rye bread—low-salt	1 slice		56	12
DINNER	steamed asparagus	2/3 cup		20	1
	boiled potato	1 medium		76	3
	sirloin steak	8 ozs.		260	57
	whole wheat bread	1 slice		56	121
	grapefruit	1/2 medium		41	1
	pear, fresh	1		122	4
	tea, herbal	8 ozs.		2	2
SNACK	potato chips	5		54	34
	☞ TOTALS (Double Check!)			1364	423
	☞ GOAL (How did you do?)				

Figure 12-2

HOW TO COUNT SODIUM MILLIGRAMS

Daily, prepare a chart like the one in Figure 12-2 that will list the item of food, size of serving, other counts (calories, etc.) and the amount of sodium you have taken. Aim for as *low* a sodium count as possible for Slimfasting results.

TYPICAL SODIUM CONTENTS OF SOME COMMON FOODS

Food	*Degree of Prep.	mg Sodium per Serving	Serving or Measure	Weight Basis
Apples	R	0.5-3.5	1 medium	3 per lb.
Apricots, fresh	R	0.9	2 medium	10 per lb.
Asparagus, spears	R	3.5	1/2 cup	2 cups cooked per lb.
Asparagus, spears, canned	O	560	1/2 cup	1 1/2 cup/14.5 oz.
Asparagus, frozen	O	1.3-12	1/2 cup	2 cups/10 oz.
Bacon, raw	O	103	1 slice	30 slices per lb.
Baking Powder, Phosphate	O	243	1 teasp.	1 teasp./2.7 g
Bananas	R	0.6-6	1 medium	3 per lb.
Beans, baked Navy and Pork	O	950	3/4 cup	1 1/2 cup/14 oz.
Beans, canned, baked	O	1130	3/4 cup	2 cups/18 oz.
Beans, w/tomato sauce	O	796	3/4 cup	1 1/2 cups/14 oz.
Beans, green	R	0.1-2.3	1/2 cup	3 cups cooked per lb.
Beans, green, canned	O	465	1/2 cup	2 cups/lb.
Beans, green, frozen	O	1.0-1.5	1/2 cup	3 cups/lb.
Beans, lima	R	0.2	1/2 cup	3 cups/lb.
Beans, lima canned	O	235	1/2 cup	3 cups/lb.
Beans, lima, frozen	O	114-235	1/2 cup	3 cups/lb.
Beef, corned	O	1850	5 oz.	
Beef, hash, corned, canned	O	610	1/2 cup	2 cups/lb.
Beef, dried	O	1220	1 oz.	
Beef, lean	R	72-92	5 oz.	
Beef, lean, Koshered	R	2270	5 oz.	
Beef, steak	R	98	5 oz.	
Beef, stew, canned	D	22	1 cup	2 cups/lb.
Beets	R	32-124	1/2 cup	2 cups/lb.
Beets, canned	O	41	1/2 cup	2 cups/lb.

*Note: R, Raw or fresh foods. O, Ordinary commercial production processes. D, Dietetic Foods

Food	Degree of Prep.	mg Sodium per Serving	Serving or Measure	Weight Basis
Beverages, alcoholic				
Beer	0	28	12 fl. oz.	—
Beer, dark	0	15	12 fl. oz.	—
Beer light	0	56	12 fl. oz.	—
Beer & ale, various	0	3.1-80	12 fl. oz.	—
Brandy	0	0.9	1 fl. oz.	—
Gin	0	.24	1 fl. oz.	—
Rum	0	0.6	1 fl. oz.	—
Whiskey, blended	0	.09	1 fl. oz.	—
Whiskey, bonded	0	.03	1 fl. oz.	—
Wine (average)	0	2.1	1 fl. oz.	—
Wine Port	0	1.2	1 fl. oz.	—
Wine Sauterne	0	3.0	1 fl. oz.	—
Beverages, carbonated*				
Coca-Cola	0	3.5-7.0	12 fl. oz.	—
Creme Soda		3.5	12 fl. oz.	—
Dr. Pepper		10.5	12 fl. oz.	—
Ginger Ale		7-28	12 fl. oz.	—
Canada Dry		63	12 fl. oz.	—
Grape Soda		42	12 fl. oz.	—
Lemon-Lime Soda		24.5	12 fl. oz.	—
Orange Crush		7	12 fl. oz.	—
Orange Soda		81	12 fl. oz.	—
Pepsi-Cola		35-49	12 fl. oz.	—

*Considerable variation may be found between bottling plants, depending upon the sodium content of the local water.

Figure 12-1 (cont'd.)

Food	Degree of Prep.	mg Sodium per Serving	Serving or Measure	Weight Basis
Root-Beer		3.5-28	12 fl. oz.	
Royal Crown Cola		17.5	12 fl. oz.	
Seven-Up		3.5	12 fl. oz.	
Strawberry Soda		17.5	12 fl. oz.	
White Rock		3.5	12 fl. oz.	
Blueberries	R	80-134	1 cup	1 cup/5 oz.
Bouillon cube, beef	O	908	1 cube	15 cubes/2 oz.
Bread, Rye & Wheat	O	112	1 slice	24 slices/lb.
Bread, White	O	112	1 thin slice	21 slices/lb.
Bread, White	O	129	1 reg. slice	18 slices/lb.
Bread, White, enriched	O	161	1 reg. slice	18 slices/lb.
Bread, Whole Wheat	O	152-211	1 slice	20 slices/lb.
Broccoli	R	11-18	3/4 cup	8 stalks/lb.
Broccoli, frozen	O	15	3/4 cup	2 cups/10 oz.
Brussels Sprouts	R	6.4-8.5	1/2 cup	2 cups/10 oz.
Brussels Sprouts, frozen	O	6.4-23	1/2 cup	2 cups/10 oz.
Butter, salted	O	42	1 pat	96 pats or teasp./lb.
Butter, sweet	O	1	1 pat	96 pats or teasp./lb.
Cabbage	R	3.2-14	1/2 cup shredded R	3 1/2 cups shredded/lb.
Cabbage		4.5-19	1/2 cup cooked	2 1/2 cups cooked/lb.
Candy				
Caramel, soft	D	16	1 pc.	50 pcs/14 oz.
Milk chocolate	O	18	1 bar-3/4 oz.	
Gum Drops	O	183	1/2 cup	2 1/2 cups/lb.
Bar, Baby Ruth	O	60	1 bar- 1 1/4 oz.	
Bar, Milky Way	O	78	1 bar- 1 1/4 oz.	

Figure 12-1 (cont'd.)

Food	Degree of Prep.	mg Sodium per Serving	Serving or Measure	Weight Basis
Carrots	R	68	1/2 cup	2 1/4 cups diced or shredded/lb.
Carrots		75	1/2 cup cooked	2 cups cooked/lb.
Carrots	O	318	1/2 cup	2 cups/lb.
Cashew nuts, roasted in oil, salted	O	226	4 oz.	
Catsup, tomato	O	204	1 tablespoon	
Celery	R	172-259	1 cup raw diced	2 1/2 cups/lb.
Celery flakes, dehyd.	O	34.5	1 tablespoon	
Celery Salt	O	672	1 teaspoon	
Celery Seed	O	3	1 teaspoon	
Cereals				
Bran, all-bran	O	340-395	1 oz.	1 pkg./1 oz.
Cornflakes	O	186	1 cup-1 oz.	1 cup/oz.
Oats, Oatmeal	R	0.2	1/4 cup uncooked	5 1/2 cups/lb.
Rice, puffed	O	.13	1/2 oz.-1 cup	2 cups/oz.
Wheat Flakes	O	367	1 cup-1 oz.	1 cup/oz.
Grape Nuts	O	186	1/4 cup-1 oz.	1/4 cup/oz.
Muffets	O	1.5	2 biscuits	24 biscuits/lb.
Puffed Wheat	O	.56	1/2 oz.-1 cup	2 cups/oz.
Shredded Wheat	O	0.5	2 biscuits	19 biscuits/lb.
Cheese, Am. Swiss	O	201	1 slice	16 slices/lb.
Cheese, Cheddar	O	173-198	1 slice	16 slices/lb.

Figure 12-1 (cont'd.)

Food	Degree of Prep.	mg Sodium per Serving	Serving or Measure	Weight Basis
Cheese, Cottage	O	330	1/2 cup	16 fl. oz./lb.
Cheese, Cream, Phila.	O	212	3 oz. pkg.	—
Cheese, Parmesan powd.	O	14.3	1 teasp.	—
Cheese, Velveeta cheese	O	910	1"x1 1/4" x 2"	—
Cherries	R	4.5	1 cup	3 cups/lb.
Cherries, sweet, dark canned	D	1.2	1/2 cup	16 fl. oz./1 lb. 1 oz.
Chicken	R	106	5 oz.	—
Chicken, light meat	R	77	5 oz.	—
Chicken, light meat breast	R	111	5 oz.	—
Chicken, dark meat	R	114	5 oz.	—
Chicken, leg meat	R	156	5 oz.	—
Chocolate syrup, Hershey	O	10.6	1 tablespoon	13 fl. oz./lb.
Cloves, whole	O	1.4	10 whole	—
Coffee, instant, Nescafe, dry	O	.84	1 teasp.	—
Coffee, reg. roasted dry	O	0.2	2 tablesp.	—
Corn, sweet	R	.15-.7	1/2 cup	—
Corn, sweet, frozen	R	65-80	1/2 cup	3 cups/lb.
Corn, sweet yellow, canned	O	252	1/2 cup	2 cups/lb.
Crackers, Graham	O	100	1 dbl. cracker	32 dbl. crackers/lb.
Crackers, Rye, Ry-Krisp	O	95	1 triple cracker	36 triple crackers/8 oz.
Crackers, Soda	O	138	1-4 pc. cracker	36 x 4 crackers/lb.
Cucumber, pickle, dill	O	318	1 pickle 1/2" dia. x 2 1/2"	—
Duck, breast	R	97	5 oz.	—
Duck, leg	R	136	5 oz.	—

Figure 12-1 (cont'd.)

174

Food	Degree of Prep.	mg Sodium per Serving	Serving or Measure	Weight Basis
Eggs, whole	R	36-62	1 med.	10 average eggs w/out shell/lb.
Frankfurters	O	610	1 med.	8/lb.
Fruit cocktail, canned in syrup	O	10	1/2 cup	2 cups/lb.
Goose, breast	R	108	5 oz.	
Goose, leg	R	136	5 oz.	
Ham, cured	O	1560	5 oz.	
Ice Cream	O	43-68	1/4 pt.	1 pt/9.5 oz.
Lamb (Lean)	R	128	5 oz.	
Lamb chop	R	129-139	5 oz.	
Lamb leg	R	111	5 oz.	
Liver, beef	R	75-492	5 oz.	
Liver, calf	R	156	5 oz.	
Liver, chicken	R	119	5 oz.	
Margarine	O	52	1 pat	96 pats or teasp./lb.
Mayonnaise	O	560	1/2 cup	2 1/2 cups/lb.
Milk, Cow's				
Milk, Condensed, sweetened	O	444	1 cup	
Milk, Evaporated	O	246	1 cup	
Milk, Whole	R	122-127	1 cup	
Mushrooms, sliced	R	3-7	1/4 cup	1 1/4 cup/lb.
Mushrooms, canned	O	283	1/4 cup	1 1/4 cup/lb.
Mustard, Prep paste	O	57	1 teasp.	
Olives, ripe pickled	O	33	1 medium	8/oz.
Olives, stuffed, pickled	O	70	1 medium	11/oz.
Onion, cooked	O	8-11	1/2 cup	2 cups/lb.
Onion Soup, cream of canned	D	72	1 cup	
Parsley flakes	O	4.4	1 tablesp.	
Parsnips	R	9-11	1/2 cup	2 cups/lb.
Peanut butter	O	16	1 tablesp.	

Figure 12-1 (cont'd.)

Food	Degree of Prep.	mg Sodium per Serving	Serving or Measure	Weight Basis
Peanuts, roasted in oil and salted	O	520	1/4 lb.	1 cup/lb.
Peas	R	1.1-9.1	1/2 cup	1 cup/lb.
Peas, frozen	O	27-295	1/2 cup	1 cup/lb.
Peas, canned, less liquor	O	306	1/2 cup	2 cups/lb.
Pea, Soup, canned	D	28-69	1 cup	
Pork, lean	R	82	5 oz.	
Pork, med. lean	R	97	5 oz.	
Pork, 10% protein	R	60	5 oz.	
Potatoes	R	7.5-9.8	1 med.	3/lb.
Potato chips	O	384	1/4 lb.	
Pretzels	O	1925	1/4 lb.	
Raisins, seedless	O	30	1 cup	3 1/4 cups/lb.
Salmon, canned	O	1190	1-7 3/4 oz. can	
Sardines, canned, various	O	424-806	1-3 3/4 oz. can	
Sauerkraut, canned	O	690	1/2 cup	2 cups/lb.
Sausage-breakfast	O	1000	1/4 lb.	
Sausage-bologna		370	1 slice	16 slices/lb.
Sausage-pork		840-870	1/4 lb. or 4 links	
Shrimp	R	159	1/4 lb.	
Spinach	R	24-165	1/2 cup	1 1/2 to 2 cups/lb.
Spinach, frozen	O	30-43	1/2 cup	3 cups/lb.
Sweet Potatoes	R	13.4	1/2 cup	2 1/2 cups/lb.
Sweet Potatoes, canned	O	66	1/2 cup	
Tomato juice	O	504	1/2 cup	
Tomato Soup, canned diluted as served	O	900	1 cup	

Figure 12-1 (cont'd.)

Food	Degree of Prep.	mg Sodium per Serving	Serving or Measure	Weight Basis
Tongue, beef	R	71-142	5 oz.	——
Tuna, canned	O	1580	7 oz. can	——
Turkey, breast	R	57	5 oz.	——
Turkey, leg meat	R	131	5 oz.	——
Veal, fillet	R	152	5 oz.	——
Veal, lean	R	68	5 oz.	——
Veal, muscle	R	163-278	5 oz.	——
Worcestershire Sauce	O	84	1 teasp.	——

Figure 12-1 (cont'd.)

177

HOW A SALT-FREE PROGRAM
DISSOLVED 80 "IMPOSSIBLE" POUNDS

Stanley MacK. was about to give up. He had 80 "impossible" pounds that refused to just "go away." He had tried other reducing plans with success, but he found it difficult to eliminate some of his favorite foods such as lamb chops, frequent cakes, pies, even ice cream. Stanley MacK. would go "wild" after a typical weight loss program and gorge himself with forbidden foods and gain back whatever had been lost. He wanted to lose his 80 "impossible" pounds but on a program that would permit him to indulge in his favorite foods, even if in moderate amounts. So a friend suggested that he follow a salt-free Slimfasting program. Here is how this easy program solved his need for eating foods and losing weight:

Set Goals. Begin by setting your weight goals. Write down your target weight. Then weigh yourself daily. Write down how much you have gained or lost. This tells you whether you are succeeding or whether you need to lower salt intake even further.

Keep a Point Scorecard. Make a copy of the sample scorecard in Figure 12-2. Set your point limits for sodium, expressed in milligrams, per day. Plan ahead each day for delicious meals within your limits. (Yes, a salt-free Slimfasting program lets you enjoy most of your favorite foods.) Keep a score each day. This helps you stay within your goal. It also helps you make certain you get your required nutrient values daily.

Throw Away Salt Shaker. This is a "must." No alternatives. No excuses. You *must* get rid of the salt shaker. You *must* get rid of all salt in your house. Do not keep any!

Be a Label Reader. On any packaged foods, read the label. Avoid any products that contain these ingredients as they would appear on the label: salt, baking powder, brine, or ingredients including sodium such as monosodium glutamate, sodium benzoate, sodium bicarbonate, sodium sulfite, sodium hydroxide, sodium cyclamate. Any label that carries the word *sodium* either alone or with another item means you should pass up that food!

Fresh Foods Preferred. Most fresh foods are rather low in sodium so they should be preferred over canned, processed or frozen ones.

Results? Stanley MacK. Becomes "Skinny." Following this simple plan, Stanley MacK. could also indulge in occasional pastries, his beloved cream-filled pies since his caloric level was *lower* and his sodium reading was very low. Now he could actually "eat his way to weight loss" on this salt-free Slimfasting program. Within five months Stanley MacK. lost almost all of the 80 "impossible" pounds. He developed a youthfully athletic physique. Friends and family noticed the change and laughingly called him "Skinny." He laughed along with them, feeling slim and great! All this and good health, through a salt-free Slimfasting program that was unbelievably easy and just as unbelievably successful!

HOW WEIGHT WAS LOST

Body cells and tissues are porous; they may be compared to a *sieve.* Salt, like sand particles, tends to absorb excess water. Carried by the bloodstream, salt becomes engorged and then clogs up the sieve-like adipose cell tissues. Compounded regularly, the salt blocks free passage of the *interstitial* and *extracellular* fluids. When the cells are blocked, they pick up and accumulate more grain-like sediment. This leads to engorgement and swelling of the cells. Like a sieve, the cells then become so filled up, fluids cannot freely pass through and cause exchanges of nutrients. Weight starts to mount up.

When you go on a salt-free Slimfasting program, the process of metabolism now draws upon the accumulated salt in your adipose fatty tissues. Your metabolism is able to dissolve, absorb and then wash out the salt from your system. It is an internal autolysis or self-digestive reaction that scrubs the cells, "reduces" them so that the sieve-like process is now possible. A clean "sieve" means a light-weight benefit. Therefore, cleansed adipose cells are light-weight. It is this simple mechanism that is able to cast out unwanted or stubborn pounds from your body.

HELPFUL HINTS FOR
SEASONING FOODS WITHOUT SALT

Under this salt-free Slimfasting program, you can enjoy seasoned foods even if salt is omitted. Here are ways to give your taste buds a tang of pleasure during Slimfasting:

1. Use lemon and lime wedges. These tart fruits are just about sodium-free and can be used freely. As a salt-substitute, try a squeeze of lemon or lime juice. You'll enjoy a fragrant, sharp flavor that makes up for the absence of salt.

2. Adventure in the world of sodium-free herbs and spices. They add a varied interest to food. Try them individually or experiment with combinations for new flavor thrills.

3. Use unsalted butter or margarine. Sprinkle with herbs for a tangy taste.

4. Avoid commercial salad dressings or mayonnaise as they may be high in sodium. Use a home made dressing of apple cider vinegar, vegetable oil and honey for the tang you love to taste on salads.

5. *Ordinary canned vegetables almost always contain sodium but the labels rarely say so.* Avoid these. Switch to home made vegetables. Season with garlic or onion powder or desired herbs and spices.

HOW TO SLIMFAST ON SALT-FREE FOODS

Advanced planning is helpful. Here are general guidelines to follow on a Slimfasting program. There aren't any foods which are totally taboo. It's basically a matter of cutting down on those which are high in salt. Here's a general guideline for Slimfasting on a salt-free program:

LOW-SALT MEATS

Lean beef, veal and lamb are fairly low in sodium. So are chicken and turkey. Processed meats, such as sausage, frankfurters, bologna and lunch meats are high. Canned meat, fish or poultry generally have added salt. Smoked meats are always high and so are ham, pork, bacon and chipped and corned beef.

Meat may be broiled, baked or boiled. The cooking process doesn't usually add to the sodium content. Cooking oils contain essentially no sodium.

LOW-SALT FISH

Fresh fish fillets, whether fresh water or ocean, are low in sodium and can be served often. The sodium content goes up in canned fish. Shellfish are high in sodium. Salted or smoked fish are higher still. Be aware that anchovies and caviar are also very high in sodium.

LOW-SALT VEGETABLES

Fresh vegetables are not only nutritionally sound but relatively low in sodium. Since salt is added during processing, many frozen, canned, dehydrated vegetables have somewhat higher sodium content.

LOW-SALT FRUITS

Fruits in any form—fresh, frozen, dried or canned—are low in sodium content and may be used freely in your menu planning.

LOW-SALT DAIRY PRODUCTS

Most dairy products are rather high in sodium. You may want to seek out salt-free dairy products in health stores or in special dairies. Low-fat dairy products are lower in sodium content.

LOW-SALT BREADS, CEREALS

With few exceptions, *natural* cereals are low in sodium. Some enriched or ready-to-serve cereals have added sodium. *Read the label!* Barley, cracked wheat, puffed wheat, shredded wheat, bran, cream of wheat, oatmeal, grits, brown rice and cornmeal are usually low in sodium. Breads are moderately high in sodium. Ask for low-salt breads and bread products such as muffins, biscuits, rolls. If a packaged product is low-salt or salt-free, it usually says so on the label.

LOW-SALT CONDIMENTS, SPICES

Many traditional condiments—ketchup, mustard, chili sauce, relishes, pickles—have high sodium content. So do barbecue sauce, soy sauce, Worcestershire sauce, bouillon cubes and canned sauces. You will do well to create your own sauce by combining apple cider vinegar, oil, honey and desired herbs.

A salt-free program will do much to help keep your adipose cell tissues clean, fresh and youthfully slim. Your entire body will enjoy better health through weight loss with a salt-free Slimfasting program. It's the unbelievably easy way to actually eat your way to a "forever slim" figure!

IN REVIEW

1. Count salt milligrams instead of calories for swift and permanent weight loss. Salt clogs up and adds weight to the billions of body adipose cell tissues. Salt is the villain in weight gain!

2. Bertha L. won the battle of lifetime overweight through a salt-free Slimfasting program. She melted her 202 pounds

and unsightly inches down to a trim 122 pounds, a neat 32 inch waistline and a size 14 dress . . . and she kept on losing more unwanted weight!

3. Plan your own salt-free Slimfasting program by following the chart listing the sodium contents of common foods. Plan to eat foods that are very low in sodium. Set your goals. Use the Practice Scorecard.

4. Stanley MacK. lost his 80 "impossible" pounds while indulging in his favorite foods on a salt-free Slimfasting program.

5. Follow the tasty hints for seasoning foods without salt.

Chapter Thirteen

Over 40?

Here are "SPC" Slimfasting Programs

to Trim "Middle Age Spread"

Folks who reach the middle years of life often do so with overweight pounds and so-called "middle age spread." With the use of an easy and tasty Sodium-Potassium-Calorie Slimfasting program (or "SPC" Slimfasting), it is possible to help wash out the accumulated weight and water and become slim and trim in the middle years. A simple "SPC" Slimfasting program can make these years the prime of your life.

MIDDLE YEARS METABOLIC SLOWDOWN

Weight gain occurs during the middle years because of a metabolic slowdown which leads to sodium-water retention and accumulated weight. In effect, it is similar to that of a *sponge*. Accumulated salt water will cause swelling. In the body, during this time of life, a little-known mineral can help counteract the effects of this sponge-like swelling that causes weight gain. The sluggish metabolism can be alerted into youthful action with the presence of this mineral: *potassium*. During a Slimfasting program with a low-sodium, high-potassium, controlled-calorie intake, you can help balance the scales so that sodium is washed out through the potassium-spurred metabolic reaction. A controlled-calorie intake further helps keep weight down. It is this *balance* that is created through an easy "SPC" Slimfasting program that can help give you a slim-trim figure in so-called "middle age" and firm up that "spread."

Sodium-Potassium Balance:
Key to Over-40 Slimness

Here is how sodium-potassium balance works within your body to keep you slim.

Sodium and potassium are similar in biological properties but different in location within your body.

Sodium is chiefly located in the fluids that circulate *outside* your adipose cell tissues and only a small amount of it is inside your cells.

Potassium is mostly *inside* the cells and a much smaller amount of it is in the body fluids.

A *balanced interrelation* of the amounts of these minerals in their different locations permits substances to pass back and forth between the sieve-like or sponge-like cells and the surrounding fluids. This process of exchange is called *osmosis.* Your metabolism must maintain a normal balance of sodium and potassium between the cells and the surrounding fluids. But during the middle years, a somewhat sluggish metabolism may not maintain this balance and an excess of sodium means that the cells absorb debris and become clogged and "heavy." Potassium may be in short supply and this can create forms of overweight. If you have a sodium problem, check with your doctor, and then follow a program that will wash out this excess in your system.

Low-Sodium, High-Potassium, Controlled-Calorie

In following an SPC Slimfasting program, begin by emphasizing or cutting down on certain foods as follows:

1. *Low-Sodium.* Plan to either cut down or eliminate foods that have high sodium counts. (See Figure 13-1 for your guideline.) Restrict or eliminate use of: salt in any form whether with your foods or as it exists in processed foods, potato chips, olives, luncheon meats, salted cheeses, salted bouillon cubes, catsup, caviar, commercial crackers, ham, herring, mustard, salted popcorn, salted salad dressings, salt pork, salted nuts, sausage, canned soups and any other foods that are salty to the taste and/or label.

2. *High-Potassium.* These include *fruits* such as raw whole apples, apricots, avocados, bananas, cantaloupes, dried dates, grapefruit, nectarines, dried cooked prunes, sun-dried raisins, orange. *Vegetables* include asparagus, all dried beans and lentils, fresh snap or green beans, Brussels sprouts, broccoli, cauliflower, corn on the cob, fresh lima beans, fresh peas, green peppers, baked or boiled potatoes, radishes, squash. *Juices* made from fresh fruits or vegetables are also prime sources of potassium.

3. *Controlled-Calorie.* Lean and fat-trimmed meats, fish, poultry, skim milk and products made from skim milk, most fresh fruits and their juices, most fresh vegetables and their juices.

YOUR "SPC" SLIMFASTING CHART

This diet chart has been prepared for people who must watch the sodium, potassium and/or calories in the food they eat. The figures are listed for average portions of food commonly eaten . . . to make it easier for you to follow your doctor's instructions.

Meat and Poultry*

	Portion	Sodium (mg.)	Potassium (mg.)	Calories
Bacon	1 strip (1 oz.)	71	16	156
Beef				
Corned Beef (canned)	3 slices	803	51	184
Hamburger	1/4 lb	41	382	224
Pot Roast (rump)	1/2 lb	43	309	188
Sirloin Steak	1/2 lb	57	545	260
Chicken (broiler)	3 1/2 oz	78	320	151
Duck	3 1/2 oz	82	285	326
Frankfurter (all beef)	1/8 lb	550	110	129
Ham				
Fresh	1/4 lb	37	260	126
Cured, butt	1/4 lb	518	239	123
Cured, shank	1/4 lb	336	155	91
Lamb				
Shoulder Chop (1)	1/2 lb	72	422	260
Rib Chop (2)	1/2 lb	68	398	238
Leg Roast	1/4 lb	41	246	96
Liver				
Beef	3 1/2 oz.	86	325	136
Calf	3 1/2 oz.	131	436	141
Pork				
Loin Chop	6 oz.	52	500	314
Spareribs (3 or 4)	3 1/2 oz.	51	360	209
Sausage (link or bulk)	3 1/2 oz.	740	140	450
Turkey	3 1/2 oz.	40	320	268
Veal				
Cutlet	6 oz.	46	448	235
Loin Chop (1)	1/2 lb.	54	384	514
Rump Roast	1/4 lb.	36	244	84

Before cooking.

Fish

	Portion	Sodium (mg.)	Potassium (mg.)	Calories
Clams (4 lg., 9 sm.)	3 1/2 oz.	36	235	82
Cod	3 1/2 oz.	70	382	78
Flounder or Sole	3 1/2 oz.	56	366	68
Lobster (1)				
Boiled, with 2 tbsp. butter	3/4 lb.	210	180	308

Figure 13-1

Oysters (5 to 8)

Fresh	3 1/2 oz.	73	121	66
Frozen	3 1/2 oz.	380	210	66
Salmon (pink, canned)	3 1/2 oz.	387	361	141
Sardines (8) Canned, in oil	3 1/2 oz.	510	560	311
Shrimp	3 1/2 oz.	140	220	91

Tuna

Canned, in oil	3 1/2 oz.	800	301	288
Canned, in water	3 1/2 oz.	41	279	127

Snacks

	Portion	Sodium (mg.)	Potassium (mg.)	Calories
Candy				
Chocolate Creams	1 candy	1	15	51
Milk Chocolate	1 oz.	30	105	152
Ice Cream				
Chocolate	1/2 pint	75	*	300
Vanilla	1/2 pint	82	210	290
Nuts				
Cashews (roasted)	6-8	2	84	84
Peanuts (roasted)				
Salted	1 tbsp.	69	105	85
Unsalted	1 tbsp.	trace	111	86
Olives				
Green	2 medium	312	7	15
Ripe	2 large	150	5	37
Potato Chips	5 chips	34	88	54
Pretzels (3 ring)	1 average	87	7	12

*Not available.

Dairy Products

	Portion	Sodium (mg.)	Potassium (mg.)	Calories
Butter (salted)	1 pat	99	2	72
Butter (unsalted)	1 pat	1	2	72
Cheese				
American, cheddar	1 oz.	197	23	112
American, processed	1 oz.	318	22	107
Cottage, creamed	3 1/2 oz	229	85	106
Cream (heavy)	1 tbsp	35	10	52
Egg	1 large	66	70	88
Milk (whole)	8 oz.	122	352	159
Oleomargarine (salted)	1 pat	99	2	72

Breads, Cereals, Etc.

	Portion	Sodium (mg.)	Potassium (mg.)	Calories
Bread				
Rye	1 slice	128	33	56
White (enriched)	1 slice	117	20	62

Figure 13-1 (cont'd.)

		Sodium	Potassium	Calories
Whole Wheat	1 slice	121	63	56
Corn Flakes	1 cup	165	40	95
Macaroni (enriched, cooked tender)	1 cup	1	85	151
Noodles (enriched, cooked)	1 cup	3	70	200
Oatmeal (cooked)	1 cup	1	130	148
Rice (white, dry)	1/4 cup	3	45	178
Spaghetti (enriched, cooked tender)	1 cup	2	92	166
Waffles (enriched)	1 waffle	356	109	209
Wheat Germ	3 tbsp	1	232	102

Beverages

	Portion	Sodium (mg.)	Potassium (mg.)	Calories
Apple Juice	6 oz.	2	187	87
Beer	8 oz.	8	46	114
Coca-Cola	6 oz.	2	88	78
Coffee (brewed)	1 cup	3	149	5
Cranberry Cocktail	7 oz.		20	130
Ginger Ale	8 oz.	18	1	80
Orange Juice				
Canned	8 oz.	3	500	120
Fresh	8 oz.	3	496	111
Prune Juice	6 oz.	4	423	138
Tea	8 oz.	2	21	2

Fruits*

	Portion	Sodium (mg.)	Potassium (mg.)	Calories
Apple	1 medium	1	165	87
Apricot				
Fresh	2-3	1	281	51
Canned (in syrup)	3 halves	1	234	86
Dried	17 halves	26	979	260
Banana	1 6-in.	1	370	85
Blueberries	1 cup	1	81	62
Cantaloupe	1/4 melon	12	251	30
Cherries				
Fresh	1/2 cup	2	191	58
Canned (in syrup)	1/2 cup	1	124	89
Dates				
Fresh	10 medium	1	648	274
Dried (pitted)	1 cup (6 oz.)	2	1150	488
Fruit Cocktail	1/2 cup	5	161	76
Grapefruit	1/2 medium	1	135	41
Grapes	22 grapes	3	158	69
Orange	1 small	1	200	49
Peaches				
Fresh	1 medium	1	202	38
Canned	2 halves, 2 tbsp. syrup	2	130	78

Figure 13-1 (cont'd.)

Pears
  Fresh.................... 1/2 pear .... 2....... 130....... 61
  Canned .... 2 halves,
                           2 tbsp. syrup..... 1....... 84....... 76
Pineapple
  Fresh.................... 3/4 cup .... 1....... 146....... 52
  Canned   1 slice and syrup.. 1....... 96....... 74
Plums
  Fresh.................... 2 medium .... 2....... 299....... 66
  Canned .... 3 medium,
                           2 tbsp. syrup..... 1....... 142....... 83
Prunes
  Dried.................... 10 large......... 8....... 694...... 255
Strawberries .... 10 large......... 1....... 164....... 37
Watermelon .... 1/2 cup......... 1....... 100....... 26

All portions weight 3 1/2 oz., unless otherwise noted.

Vegetables*

	Portion	Sodium (mg.)	Potassium (mg.)	Calories
Artichoke				
Base and soft end of leaves ..	1 large bud	30.......	301	44
Asparagus				
Fresh	2/3 cup	1.......	183.......	20
Canned	6 spears.........	271.......	191.......	21
Beans, baked	5/8 cup	2.......	704.......	159
Beans, green				
Fresh	1 cup	5.......	189.......	31
Canned	1 cup	295.......	109.......	30
Beans, lima				
Fresh....................	5/8 cup	1.......	422........	111
Canned	1/2 cup.........	271.......	255.......	110
Frozen	5/8 cup	129.......	394.......	118
Beets				
Fresh....................	1/2 cup.........	36.......	172.......	27
Canned	1/2 cup.........	196.......	138.......	31
Broccoli				
Fresh....................	2/3 cup.........	10.......	267.......	26
Brussels Sprouts	6-7 medium......	10.......	273.......	36
Cabbage				
Raw, shredded............	1 cup	20.......	233.......	24
Cooked	3/5 cup.........	14.......	163.......	20
Carrots				
Raw.....................	1 large.........	47.......	341.......	42
Cooked	2/3 cup.........	33.......	222.......	31
Canned	2/3 cup.........	236.......	120.......	30
Cauliflower	7/8 cup.........	9.......	206.......	22
Celery....................	1 outer, 3 inner stalks	63.......	170.......	8
Corn				
Fresh....................	1 medium ear	trace......	196.......	100
Canned	1/2 cup	196.......	81......	70
Cucumber, pared	1/2 medium	3.......	80.......	7
Lettuce, iceberg	3 1/2 oz.........	9	264.......	14

Figure 13-1 (cont'd.)

Mushrooms				
(uncooked)	10 sm., 4 lg......	15.......	414.......	28
Onions (uncooked)..........	1 medium.......	10.......	157.......	38
Peas				
Fresh	2/3 cup.........	1.......	196.......	71
Canned	3/4 cup.........	236.......	96.......	88
Frozen	3 1/2 oz.........	115.......	135.......	68
Potatoes				
Boiled (in skin)	1 medium.......	3.......	407.......	76
French Fried	10 pieces........	3.......	427.......	137
Radishes..................	10 small	18.......	322.......	17
Sauerkraut	2/3 cup..........	747.......	140.......	18
Spinach	1/2 cup.........	45.......	291.......	21
Tomatoes				
Raw....................	1 medium.......	4.......	366.......	33
Canned	1/2 cup.........	130.......	217.......	21
Paste	3 1/2 oz.........	38.......	888.......	82

Note: Because vegetable counts vary greatly from raw to cooked state, values are for cooked vegetables with no added salt unless otherwise noted. Frozen vegetables have virtually the same count as fresh vegetables, when cooked, unless otherwise noted.

Figure 13-1 (cont'd.)

HOW AN "SPC" SLIMFASTING PROGRAM TURNED "MIDDLE AGE SPREAD" INTO AN HOURGLASS FIGURE

Stella DeB. was ashamed of her "middle age spread." She would waddle instead of walk, expand when sitting instead of being trim. She had tried some reducing programs but could not get rid of the bulges that seemed to balloon her out of all proportions. No matter what she tried, the heavy hanging embarrassing bulges still clung to her body. She wanted to do anything to get rid of the so-called "middle age spread." So it was that she followed an easy "SPC" Slimfasting program as follows:

Set Your Goals in Advance

Decide how many milligrams of sodium, potassium and how many calories you will take in daily. Stella DeB. set these goals in advance:

500   milligrams of sodium daily (or less) but no higher.

2500   milligrams of potassium daily (or more) but not less.

1500   calories daily (or less) but no higher.

Keep Simple Score: Consult the "SPC" Slimfasting chart in this chapter for your counts. Keep a simple daily score of selected foods. This tells you how you are progressing and whether you need to make any adjustments. Do not cheat! You'll only be fooling yourself.

Weigh Yourself Daily: If the scales go *up,* it means you need to make some adjustments. Lower sodium intake. Increase potassium intake. Control or lower caloric intake. If the scales go *down,* it means the internal balance is taking place and you continue on.

Tape Measure Yourself Daily: Keep an accurate record to see if your inches (and bulges) are going down. If they do not, then you need to lower sodium intake even further, while increasing potassium and controlling caloric intake.

Basic "SPC" Slimfasting Program

First Three Days: A wide variety of fresh fruits and their juices. Eat and drink as much as desired. *Benefit:* The very low sodium and very high potassium count helps mineralize your cells and wash out accumulated debris. The *high concentration of potassium* that can work freely during Slimfasting *without interference* of other foods gives it dynamic cell-washing power.

Fourth-Fifth-Sixth Days: A wide variety of fresh fruits and vegetables and their juices. Eat and drink as much as desired. Now add smaller portions of lean meat or poultry and some skim milk products. Select ONLY those that are low in sodium. *Benefit:* You are now helping to balance the scales with a higher potassium and lower sodium intake through these varieties of foods.

Seventh-Eighth-Ninth Days: Select only those fruits, vegetables, juices that are low in calories, although high in potassium. Follow the same rule with meats, fish, grains. Always trim away all visible fat.

Important: You MUST stick to your agreed-upon sodium-potassium-calorie goals. You MUST remain within these limits if you want Slimfasting to succeed. As stated above, if you cheat, you will only be fooling yourself.

POUNDS WASH OUT, INCHES SHRINK DOWN

Stella DeB. saw the pounds literally wash right out of her body under this "SPC" Slimfasting program. Her daily weigh-in and tape measuring told her the wonderful truth: She was slimming down by leaps and bounds! By the end of the ninth day, she saw her spreading girth shrink down, her over-ample bust become slimmer, her heavy thighs become firmer. She continued on this "SPC" program for the rest of the month in the easy 3-day cycles. Soon, Stella DeB. was down to a svelte 120 pounds. Exhilarated, she had to buy herself a whole new wardrobe. She now boasted that, thanks to "SPC" Slimfasting, her "middle age spread" had been transformed into an hourglass figure! Now she follows the basics of a low-sodium, high-potassium, controlled-calorie program and she is able to keep her slim and youthful shape!

HOW "SPC" SLIMFASTING ADJUSTS BODY SCALES

Picture your body with a built-in scale. Metabolism maintains a balance between sodium and potassium. But during middle years, a sluggish metabolism cannot maintain this balance of your internal scale. Therefore, an excess of sodium tips the scales *against* your favor. To correct this metabolic weakness, you need to alert it by an intake of high potassium foods. This mineral can now help wash out accumulated sodium and thereby tip the scales *in* your favor.

Potassium keeps your cells slim. Sodium is a mischief maker from the surrounding fluid. A potassium deficiency "opens the gateway" and the sodium mischief-maker barges into the cell. Sodium has a "magnetic" action and attracts particles that build up weight. Furthermore, an excess of sodium alters the acid-alkaline balance (pH) of the cell, creating a toxic condition that causes the formation of necrotic (dead) tissue which blocks the sieve-like wall and acts as a cement. This accumulates and weight is built up. Since you have billions upon billions of adipose cell tissues, this imbalance can create tremendous overweight. It is potassium that is needed to act as a *dynamic cell-cleanser* to wash out the weighty sodium and thereby create slimness.

FASTING CREATES THIS ACTION

Your metabolism can create this delicate balance if it can work *without competition* from intake of most other foods. Therefore, when you devote three days to a high potassium program, your metabolism is free from the obligation of working upon fats, proteins, carbohydrates and other elements; instead, your metabolism can now devote full attention to using potassium for this cell-cleansing response. A simple Slimfasting can create this weight-losing response.

Taking Diuretics? Boost Potassium Intake

John A. took a diuretic, that is, a chemical that would take out sodium from the system. Since he was in his middle years, his sluggish metabolism had upset his internal sodium-potassium "scale" and his adipose cell tissues had accumulated the sludge that gave him a shameful "bay window" as well as some 70 overweight pounds. John A. knew he had to wash out the sodium from his body and the chemical diuretic was supposed to do it. Yet, he still had his heavy weight and felt simultaneously weak, dizzy, nervous. Something was wrong.

DIURETIC CREATES SODIUM-POTASSIUM LOSS

John A.'s problem was common to those who took a diuretic. Namely, the diuretic also washes out needed potassium from the system. The kidney function does not differentiate between sodium and potassium. He lost much sodium, but with it, needed potassium. As a result, his overweight and "bay window" changed slightly because a potassium deficiency meant his cell-cloggings could not be washed out. It was a vicious cycle.

HEALTH PROBLEMS

John A., like others who take diuretics, suffers the consequences of a potassium loss. There was a reaction of vertigo (dizziness or loss of balance), heartbeat irregularities. Also, he had a feeling of weakness in his muscular contractions. John A. had to make some changes in his methods of weight loss.

SIMPLE ONCE-A-MONTH "SPC" SLIMFASTING PROGRAM

John A. needed to boost his potassium intake, reduce his sodium intake and caloric count. He did this on a simple program:

During the first seven days of each month, he went on a simple "SPC" Slimfasting program. The first two days were devoted to high potassium foods with low sodium intake. The next two days were devoted to low sodium foods with only minor emphasis upon potassium and calories. The final three days were devoted to low-sodium, high-potassium and low-calorie foods. He made his selection from a chart such as the one in this chapter.

NATURAL DIURETIC, HEALTHY
WEIGHT LOSS, YOUTHFUL REWARD

Even though the "SPC" Slimfasting program acted as a natural diuretic, the high potassium intake meant he was no longer dizzy, his heart and muscles were healthy and, most important, he began to lose much of his bay window. The daily weigh-in showed pound after pound being washed out of his system. He went through three of these Once-A-Month SPC Slimfasting programs until he found that his waistline measured a neat 34, his weight was a youthful 145, his health was bubbling over with vital energy—and he was well over the 50-year age line. Now John A. follows this easy Once-A-Month SPC Slimfasting program and maintains his slim weight. The rest of the month he is careful to count sodium-potassium-calories to keep his internal "scale" balanced in his favor. He looks to nature for diuretic foods and healthy weight loss.

How a Potassium Slimfasting Program
Melts "Middle Age Spread"

Basically, potassium is a "reducing mineral" that is defined as an *electrolyte*. That is, a substance that is transformed into *ions* or an activator through metabolism. When potassium enters your system, the methods of metabolism transform it into an activator which then performs as a conductor of electricity. It carries a positive charge. It is empowered to flow through your miles of bloodstream and then to electronically charge your cells through the means of an ultrasonic sound-type of cleansing.

SODIUM VS. POTASSIUM

Sodium is a substance that is also taken up by the body through metabolism and then transformed into a form so that it will cling to the billions of body cells and tissues. It is potassium that is then needed to enter the intracellular, extracellular and plasma fluids to perform the electrolyte or ultrasonic sound action whereby the cells are cleansed of the accumulated sodium sediment that clings to the sieve-like walls. It is potassium that is needed to wash and bathe the cells. But if there is an abundance or oversupply of sodium, then potassium is the "loser" in this battle. Sodium, as the winner, clogs up more and more cells and weight gain occurs. A balance is needed!

BENEFITS OF BALANCE

During a Slimfasting program, a higher amount of potassium enables your body to use its electrolyte power to cell-cleanse and reduce quantity of sediment. It is important for potassium to work *without interference* of other nutrients. That is why a Slimfasting program will give you the best benefits. If you eat high-potassium foods with a regular eating program, your metabolism must accommodate the potassium and the other nutrients from other foods. This dilutes and reduces the working power of potassium. When you Slimfast, focussing upon high-potassium foods, then your metabolism is free to work solely upon this mineral which it then can transform full force into an electrolyte which is used as an electronic activator to slim down your water-logged tissues.

Liquids become absorbed in sodium and weight then builds up. This is a form of edema which causes so-called "middle age spread." Your body needs potassium to wash out your sodium along with accumulated liquids and thereby reduce the "spare tire" or "inches" that are the bane of middle age folks. This can be most effectively accomplished during a simple Sodium-Potassium-Calorie Slimfasting program.

During the time of sluggish metabolism of middle years, sodium shows an affinity for liquids in the cells. It has the effect of increasing the volume of extracellular fluids, including blood plasma. To distribute this increased blood volume, the heart now must work more vigorously. This creates a strain on the bloodstream, the vascular system and predisposes you to hypertension and heart trouble, associated ailments with overweight. Therefore, the key would be to reduce sodium content, boost potassium intake, control caloric amounts. Control the osmotic rhythm through SPC Slimfasting and the middle years can be slim years that offer the hope for many, many more decades of youthful health!

SUMMARY

1. Middle years metabolic slowdown means increased sodium retention and water-logged tissues such as in edema. This creates "middle age spread."

2. A sodium-potassium balance through Slimfasting helps create better osmosis or exchange of substances so that cells are not overburdened and weighty.

3. It's easy to follow the SPC Slimfasting program with the charts.

4. Stella DeB. turned "middle age spread" into an hourglass figure by following an easy 9-day SPC Slimfasting program.

5. SPC Slimfasting adjusts body scales for a sodium-potassium balance.

6. John A. used "natural diuretics" for better weight loss. His "bay window" was soon a slim 34 inch waistline. Reducing was fun!

7. With a potassium Slimfasting program, an alerted metabolism keeps cells free of edema (sodium-swollen water) and promotes youthful slimness.

Chapter Fourteen

Fifteen Slimfasting Programs
for Quick-Easy Weight Loss

Fasting is NOT starvation! It is a planned *reduction* and *limitation* and *selection* of certain foods. On a Slimfasting program, you decide upon certain foods or categories of foods that will make up your total dietary intake. This helps keep you physically and mentally active while pounds and inches just fade away. You also continue taking in foods, even if limited and in smaller amounts, so you do not go hungry while you lose weight.

SLIMFASTING STIMULATES QUICK-EASY WEIGHT LOSS

Under your selected Slimfasting program, your metabolism is alerted to devote almost *total* activity upon the stored up fat, carbohydrates, calories in your system. This creates an active metabolism so that stubborn or unwanted pounds and inches are taken right out of your body, quickly and easily and, even more important, permanently. For example, to lose one pound of fat, you must burn up 3500 more calories than you consume. If you have a sedentary lifestyle, you burn up even less than 3500 calories in a day. It would be difficult, under ordinary reducing plans, to lose even one pound a day unless you can continuously burn up 3500 calories. Under Slimfasting, the restriction of food creates a metabolic reaction whereby you may lose about five pounds the very first day or *20 pounds over a weekend!*

THE WEIGHT-MELTING POWER OF SLIMFASTING

When you select a Slimfasting program, it calls for an adequate amount of food to keep you feeling fit and "filled up." But because the amounts are less than your normal intake, you start to lose weight almost immediately. Since your body is almost all water, Slimfasting acts by liquefying stored up fat, carbohydrates, calories, and literally washing them right out of your system. (If you weigh 165 pounds, you consist of about 100 pounds of water.) Much water retention is traced to an accumulation of cell-clogging sodium. Under any of the following Slimfasting programs, the tasty sodium-free or sodium-low items enable your metabolic reactions to loosen and then wash out the sodium from your system. This creates quick-easy weight loss—while you continue eating! Basically, the limitation of food intake is the technique that permits your metabolic responses to work *without interference* upon your stored up fat, carbohydrates, calories and "burn" them right out of your body! Once these weighty substances have been washed out of your body, your system then starts to live off your stored up reserves. Any excesses are further depleted to create even more dramatic and welcome weight loss. All this is done with little or no effort on your part. It's the quick and easy way to lose unwanted pounds and inches.

HOW TO FOLLOW YOUR SLIMFASTING PROGRAM

Here's a simple guide to help you follow your Slimfasting program:

1. Decide how many pounds you want to lose. Write down your goal. Then keep a chart. Daily, weigh yourself to see how you are succeeding. This helps give you emotional incentive to continue.

2. When you select your Slimfasting program, resolve NOT to cheat. To do so means you will not lose unwanted pounds. Be honest with yourself. Decide you will stick to the Slimfasting program.

3. Schedule your Slimfasting program on your calendar. Whether for two days, four days or longer, you should mark down your schedule and follow it faithfully.

4. The day before your first Slimfasting day, eat modestly. Drink lots of liquids. Prepare your system for the Slimfasting program.

5. During your Slimfasting, continue with your regular routine. Take a positive attitude. Mentally focus your thoughts on weight loss. Your attitude should be that you will continue with Slimfasting because you want to lose pounds and inches.

6. If you wish, Slimfast with a friend. This makes it more fun.

7. You will notice that as wastes are eliminated, you will have improved body tone as well as better mental response. You will feel more youthful.

8. To break your fast, *do it gently*. On the first day at your Slimfasting end, do NOT use salt in any form. Drink lots of water, at least a quart a day. As you resume other foods, eat them slowly, chew them very carefully. Do not over-burden your digestive system that has been cleansed and purified through Slimfasting. Do it very slowly and gently.

9. As you ease into your regular eating schedule, be sure to use lots of fresh fruits and vegetables and their juices to li-quefy your system. Try not to overeat at any time, under any circumstances.

10. During any Slimfasting program, follow these health hints: Keep yourself warm, enjoy lots of fresh air, avoid drinking stimulating beverages such as coffee, tea (except herbal tea), soft drinks, alcohol. Do not smoke. Take daily showers or baths to help your body pores wash out stored up toxins. Bathwater should be warm. Avoid hot or cold baths of any sort. Do not make any jerky or sudden move-ments since this may make you dizzy. Be sure to get a good night's sleep every night during Slimfasting.

Now, here is a selection of 15 Slimfasting programs to make weight loss a tasty, delicious and exciting occasion.

#1—BROWN RICE AND FRUIT

Eat as much steamed brown rice and fruit as you prefer throughout the program. With a wide variety of fruit available, each dish of brown rice can taste different. This is ideal for losing weight gained during a vacation cruise or at a holiday resort.

It was used by vacationing Arlene LaD. who had gained un-sightly pounds and bulgy inches during a long ocean voyage cruise where she could not resist endless varieties of available foods. Back home, she found that her clothes were too tight, her weight scale "screamed" her added pounds. To lose weight quickly and easily, she followed a brown rice and fruit diet for five days. *Results?* Stored fats and calories were burned up and she shed those unwanted pounds and inches. Soon she was slimmer than before the cruise. Also, the brown rice filled her up so she felt no hunger while pound after pound and inch after inch just "vanished" from her body! It was the most amazing reducing plan she ever tried.

#2—BROWN RICE AND VEGETABLES

Eat all the brown rice and either raw or slightly cooked vegetables you want. Since vegetables are very low in calories and carbohydrates, you will lose very quickly.

#3—GRAPEFRUIT AND LEAN MEAT

Begin each of your daily meals with a large, raw grapefruit. Section it. Chew the sections and swallow them slowly. Then you may have a small portion of any desired very lean and fat-trimmed meat.

#4—THE ALL FRUIT FAST

Eat all the fresh raw fruit that you wish, in any amounts, either as three meals or as six meals.

#5—THE ALL VEGETABLE FAST

Eat all the fresh raw vegetables that you wish, in any amounts, either as three meals or as six meals.

#6—RAW FRUIT JUICES

Throughout the day, drink all the fresh raw fruit juices that you wish. Enjoy them singly or in combination, according to your tastes.

#7—RAW VEGETABLE JUICES

Throughout the day, drink all the fresh raw vegetable juices that you wish. Enjoy them singly or in combination, according to your tastes.

#8—A DAIRY FAST

Emphasize skim milk products only. It was this fasting program that helped Ralph N. lose some 39 unwanted pounds. He would devote the first half of the fasting day to drinking skim milk (flavor with such spices as cinnamon, dill seed, ginger, mint, even parsley flakes). Ralph N. devoted the second half of the fasting day to more solid cheeses such as cottage, farmer or pot cheese. He would occasionally have sliced Muenster or Swiss if it was of a natural and salt-free source. A nightcap would be a glass of skim milk flavored with a bit of vanilla. Rewards? In the short time of two months, Ralph N. had lost his 39 unwanted pounds. This Slimfasting program created weight loss because of the alkaline reaction in the system. Acidosis can be diluted with the alkaline reaction and thereby be washed out of the system. This creates a mobilization of detoxifying reaction responses that neutralize the toxins. Calcium in the milk helps the bloodstream maintain a more constant pH (acid level) reading and this helps cellular washing for better weight loss. This easy dairy fast helped Ralph N. lose the unwanted pounds. They were lost forever!

#9—SKIM MILK AND BANANAS

In combination, they offer good taste as well as dramatic and swift weight loss. The vitamins and minerals of the skim milk activate properties in the banana to alkalize the gastrointestinal tract; this helps coat the digestive tract and thereby ease appetite urge and also promote better weight loss through cellular slimming.

#10—EGG-ORANGE COMBINATION

Limit yourself to 1 egg per day with a wide variety of different oranges. Try them in sections, in a blenderized puree, eating out of the rind. The enzymes in the orange will use the protein from the egg to alert your metabolism to loosen and dissolve accumulated weighty substances.

#11—STRAWBERRY AND YOGURT PROGRAM

Schedule three cups of yogurt daily into which you stir a portion of strawberries. (Tip: Use desired herbs and spices to add zest and taste.) The raw fruit minerals will be used by the vitamins from the milk to help metabolize accumulated wastes and then wash them out of your system.

#12—BRAN AND CHEESE

Select any skim milk cheeses you desire. Eat with bran in the form of three daily meals. Again, you can add new taste to each dish by the addition of any desired herbs or spices. The bran acts as a natural appetite depressant by absorbing minerals from the cheeses and "swelling up" during digestion to give you a feeling of satisfaction. The bran also creates swifter transit time; this means, it does not remain too long in your digestive tract so it does not add much weight. Instead, it "scrubs" your tract and helps take along added substances. The skim milk cheeses add an alkaline reaction to combat acidosis.

#13—RAW SALADS

Create any desired raw chewy salads that you flavor with a sprinkle of lemon or lime juice and a dollop of skim milk cottage cheese. Chew and eat the salads, divided into three or five daily meals. Prepared as a salad, you have the satiety-response of having eaten a chewy meal. Low calorie salads are important. They contain important vitamins, minerals and enzymes which are used by your metabolic system to loosen up and then wash out accumulated cellular debris and help create weight loss.

#14—FISH AND VEGETABLES

Select desired fish from deep waters (avoid shellfish which are high in calories and from polluted shores) and eat either baked or broiled, twice daily. Eat each fish meal with an assortment of fresh raw vegetables which are prime sources of enzymes that will take the polyunsaturated fatty acids of fish and use them to wash and cleanse the adipose cell tissues.

#15—CHICKEN AND FRUIT

Lean cuts of white chicken are good sources of protein which can be taken up by the vitamins of the fruit to activate your metabolism and cause an improved metabolic response that is comparable to spontaneous combustion. This creates "burning" of substances and dramatic weight loss.

Depending upon your individual tastes and circumstances, you can vary these Slimfasting programs. They can offer you an endless variety of taste thrills that make losing weight a delightful experience.

GENERAL GUIDELINES FOR SLIMFASTING

1. Once you select your Slimfasting program, decide that you will remain with it throughout the agreed-upon time span. When you emotionally attune yourself to the program and its weight loss, you will physically relate to it.

2. For very heavy overweight that you want to lose speedily, select a "liquid only" Slimfasting program. Without solid food, your metabolism can work "full force" to rid your body of unwanted and burdensome weight.

3. To ease the reaction of hunger pains, use natural, unprocessed bran with your program. Use one tablespoon in a juice, three times daily. Use one tablespoon over a raw fruit or vegetable platter. Sprinkle bran over other foods. The bran has a cellulose-expansion reaction that eases hunger pains during weight loss.

4. If you feel an uncontrollable appetite urge, then select a "liquids only" Slimfasting program with bran. This helps wash out debris and burdensome weight from your body without making you feel hungry. The bran is able to soothe your desire to eat.

5. If you have anxious taste buds, soothe your tongue and appetite with a warm liquid Slimfasting program. That is,

prepare *clear* broth, bouillon, consomme and take three servings daily. But remember, *no salt* of any kind! This warm liquid, sipped slowly, eases appetite urge and makes you feel comfortably full as pounds and inches slip away.

6. On any Slimfasting program, it is important to drink lots and lots of water, an hour before a meal, an hour afterward and regularly throughout the day. It is important to thoroughly *hydrate* your system so that the end products (burdensome weight debris) can be washed out through your eliminative channels. Also, water helps make you feel filled up. It's calorie free, too!

7. For most cooked foods on your Slimfasting program, be sure to cook thoroughly. That is, all meat foods should be cooked as long as possible without burning. The reason is that longer cooking tends to reduce the amount of fats, calories, and carbohydrates. (Plant foods such as vegetables, already low in calories and carbohydrates, should be eaten raw to preserve enzymes and nutrients or steamed slightly to make more palatable.)

8. For any chewy foods, be sure to chew very, very thoroughly. Make a ritual out of it. This gives you appetite satisfaction and also improves your metabolic fat-melting response.

9. For any liquid program, make a ritual out of the drinking. Sip slowly, savor the liquid in your mouth, enjoy its fragrance, then swallow slowly. Wait a moment or two, then follow through with another ritualized sip-savor-swallow routine. This will make you feel totally satisfied and also boost metabolic reactions for better weight loss.

10. Daily, take a brisk 45 minute walk in the early part of the morning and at twilight. This helps keep you refreshed and alert.

Fasting is the planned, no-fuss, no-starvation way to promote quick-easy weight loss. You have a variety of different tasty Slimfasting programs at your disposal. It makes reducing a joyful experience!

MOST IMPORTANT

1. Slimfasting offers quick-easy weight loss through better metabolic reaction and spontaneous combustion of burdensome fats.

2. Before you begin, follow the 10-step Slimfasting program.

3. Arlene LaD. lost bulky pounds and inches accumulated during a feasting cruise through a simple weekend Slimfasting program.

4. On a dairy fast, Ralph N. lost 39 unwanted pounds in jiffy time.

5. Select any of the 15 available Slimfasting programs for your own needs.

6. Be rewarded with "no fault" weight loss when following the ten general guidelines.

Chapter Fifteen

How Slimfasting Re-Adjusts

Weight-Losing Hormone "Clocks"

Two "biological clocks" in your body control the amount of weight you put on and take off. With proper adjustment, you can control these "clocks" so that you can take off excessive pounds and inches. With Slimfasting, you can "balance" the delicate "mainsprings" of these "clocks" so they release a steady amount of "ticking" to keep you youthfully slim. Slimfasting gives you control over these "clocks" so that you can maintain a desired weight and become "forever slim."

PITUITARY GLAND—WEIGHT CONTROLLING "BIOLOGICAL CLOCK"

Called the "master gland" of the body, it issues a set of hormones that can give you excessive weight as well as inches. The pituitary gland, about the size of a pea, hangs from a short stalk at the base of the brain. Very tiny, it contains three lobes which secrete at least nine known hormones. It also participates in many complex functions that influence your health. The pituitary also houses a little-known substance called the "appestat" which is the appetite-controlling center of your brain. With proper Slimfasting techniques, this "appestat" can be soothed so that you do not feel any uncontrollable and unhealthy eating urges.

WEIGHT-CONTROLLING HORMONE
SENT INTO BLOODSTREAM

A properly balanced "pituitary clock" will send forth a supply of important hormones into the bloodstream that tend to influence weight levels. An imbalanced pituitary will send spurious hormones that may cause unhealthy, rapid and stubborn weight gain. For serious problems, see your family physician.

ANTERIOR PITUITARY INFLUENCES WEIGHT

The anterior, or front part of the pituitary, secretes hormones that are then able to influence the way carbohydrates (sugars and starches) are metabolized and "burned" in the body. A deficiency of anterior pituitary hormones means that these weight-causing substances will remain stored in the body and weight gain then follows.

POSTERIOR PITUITARY BURNS UP SUGAR

The posterior, or back part of the pituitary, secretes the *pitressin* and *pittocin* hormones which focus specifically upon digestive metabolism of sugar. These two hormones need to be available in a steady supply, like the ticking of a clock, so that ingested sugar can then be "burned up" and washed out of the body through the bloodstream. If there is a deficiency of either the *pitressin* or *pittocin* hormones (often, both are so involved that they work together and cannot be separated), then sugar is improperly burned and pounds and inches start to accumulate.

HOW SLIMFASTING "WINDS UP" AND "ADJUSTS" HORMONE CLOCKS

A Slimfasting program that zeroes in on the pituitary gland, supplying it with nutrients that will "wind up" the "mainspring" and "adjust" the clock so that the "ticking" or hormone supply is made available to the body, will help metabolize and burn up accumulated sugars and starches.

Feed your pituitary with a strong supply of vitamins A and C and iron and it can then function adequately. In particular, it is helpful to go on a Slimfasting program emphasizing these nutrients alone so that the pituitary can be nourished without having to share with other body parts and therefore be "adjusted" so it can issue important carbohydrate-burning hormones.

The Simple Fruit That Stimulates Calorie-Burning Hormones

A simple, delicious, everyday fruit contains the needed vitamins and the mineral that acts as an energizer for the pituitary and stimulates it to "tick" forth a steady supply of calorie-burning hormones.

The fruit is the grape. Specifically, the *black grape* is an all-natural food for the calorie-burning pituitary hormones.

CALORIE-DESTROYING SUBSTANCE

Black grapes contain a protein or amino acid called *oenocyanine* which acts as an electric charge in the bloodstream. When you eat a portion of black grapes or drink their freshly prepared juice, your digestive system takes the *oenocyanine,* combines it with the fruit's vitamins A and C and iron and transports it through your bloodstream to the pituitary gland. Here the posterior or back part of the gland receives it eagerly and uses it as "electronic energy" to stimulate the "mainspring" so that there is a secretion of the needed calorie-melting *pitressin* and *pittocin* hormones. These hormones are powerful. They have unique sugar-splitting and starch-splitting powers. They can help destroy accumulated weights caused by car-bohydrates. They can actually destroy calories from your billions of adipose cell tissues. This is made possible when your metabolism uses the *oenocyanine* and nutrients to activate the gland and send forth the needed carbohydrate-dissolving hormones.

Three Day Grape Juice Slimfasting
Washes away Unsightly Pounds

Anna S. wanted to get rid of her unsightly pounds in time for an approaching high school class reunion. She wanted to do it quickly. She had tried other methods but as soon as the pounds went off, they came right back on. She knew there was something amiss with her metabolism and wanted a program that was swift, simple, successful in getting rid of those 48 unwanted, unsightly, and unattractive pounds. Anna S. did not want her former classmates to see how fat she had become throughout the years. So she went on a simple three day grape juice Slimfasting program. Here is what she did:

For three days, she drank as much grape juice as she desired, preferably from black grapes and home squeezed. In between, she drank as much water as she desired. She also kept herself physically active, took daily needle spray tepid showers, obtained nightly rest. Anna S. frequently ate a plate of the black grapes to give herself chewing satisfaction.

POUND-AFTER-POUND WASHES AWAY

Amazed, Anna S. saw how pound-after-pound just washed away. Her daily weigh-in told her the happy truth. The stubborn weight was melting right out of her body. By the end of the third day, she had lost much of her undesired weight.

CONTINUES GRAPE PROGRAM FOR REST OF WEEK

Anna S. *slowly* eased out of her fast with a return to other foods in moderate amounts. But she continued with her grape program. Daily, she would eat a bunch of grapes for dessert after each of her meals. Daily, she would drink one glass of black grape juice *before* breakfast, *before* her noon meal and *before* her main evening meal. She followed this program for the rest of the week. Basically, she had a Three Day Grape Juice Slimfasting program and then a four day moderate food intake with raw grapes and their juices. It was all over within one short week.

SCALES SHOW 48-POUND LOSS

Happily, Anna S. leaped for joy when she saw that the 48 stubborn pounds were lost after only 27 days. Her daily weigh-in was a cause for much celebration. Not only that, her formerly "matronly fat" shape had now slimmed down into a lovely silhouette. She most certainly did celebrate at the high school class reunion where everybody remarked how young and slim she looked and that she "hadn't changed a bit" over the years.

To keep slim, Anna S. follows a once-a-month grape juice Slimfasting program for three days. She also finds her appetite has reduced so she eats but does not overeat.

THE CALORIE-DESTROYING POWER OF
THE THREE DAY GRAPE JUICE SLIMFASTING PROGRAM

The substance *oenocyanine* is energized by vitamins and minerals in the grape to nourish the pituitary. During Slimfasting, the forces of the body are released from the burden of food digestion. Instead, these forces are now *fully concentrated* upon the *oenocyanine* and nutrients of the grape. These forces propel them via the bloodstream to the anterior (front) and posterior (back) segments of the pituitary gland. Here, the gland takes these nutrients, uses them to alert the secretion of the *pitressin* and *pittocin* hormones so that they can burn up accumulated carbohydrates and calories.

In effect, during Slimfasting, these nutrients actually "wind up" the hormone clocks and enable them to "tick" steadily to burn up weight!

More Benefits: During a Slimfasting program of black grapes, the hormones are used to burn up unwanted fatty deposits, along with huge quantities of impurities embedded within them. This creates a healthful form of internal cleansing and detoxification. The alerted *pitressin* and *pittocin* hormones alert the metabolism to "burn" the expendable fat and damaged tissues while vital and healthy tissues are left intact and nourished. The result is that the entire body responds. There is a cleansing action as the hormones promote the expulsion of toxins and metabolic wastes with speed and efficiency. This internal miracle is possible when the digestive system is relieved of the burden of handling food and can focus and target its attention on using the elements of the black grapes for the pituitary gland.

Slimfasting Programs for Pituitary Gland Weight Melting

Activate your "biological clock" so it will secrete more "ticking" hormones that melt away accumulated calories, carbohydrates and other weight with regular Slimfasting programs. You can nourish this "master gland" with a variety of different foods that act as fuel to its mainspring within your brain. Here are some suggested Slimfasting programs that zero in on alerting your pituitary gland:

Cooked Grains. Whole grain oats, cornmeal, barley, wheat are prime sources of vitamins as well as iron. When your digestive system receives these grains, it transports these nutrients via the bloodstream to the pituitary. This gland then uses the needed vitamins and iron to activate the secretion of the important weight melting hormones. A 3-day whole grain Slimfasting program keeps you filled up while your hormone clock triggers off a steady weight loss.

Raw Berry Program. Select seasonal berries that can be eaten raw such as blueberries, strawberries, gooseberries, blackberries, loganberries and others. This is a "mono-diet" which *concentrates* solely upon the vitamins and plant iron in the berries. Without interference, your digestive system can now work to capacity in transporting these nutrients to your pituitary to energize this "clock" to tick forth regular weight-destroying factors. Eat the berries singly or in combination. If you prefer, add a little bit of honey and skim milk for more flavor.

Chewy Nut Program. Supply yourself with a variety of different available nuts. These include filberts, shelled walnut meats, peanuts and others. You may also include shelled almonds. Chew them very thoroughly. For two days, subsist on these nuts. They are a powerhouse of good nut vitamins and iron that offer an input to the pituitary so it can use them for better hormone secretion and fat melting powers.

Chewy Seed Program. For two days, Slimfast solely on sunflower seeds and any other available seeds. Be sure to chew very thoroughly. Seeds are a prime source of nature-created nutrients that will be used by your pituitary for better hormone secretion. Drink lots of water throughout the day to provide a moist vehicle by which these nutrients can be transported to the pituitary.

Citrus Fruit Program. Select a variety of seasonal citrus fruits that are to be *eaten.* Oranges, grapefruits, tangerines, lemon-lime wedges (in moderation). Make a fruit compote and drizzle with a bit of honey. Eat these fruits for several days. They are a prime source of needed vitamins and minerals that are tonics to the pituitary and enter into the components of the calorie-burning hormones.

It is important to keep your pituitary clock ticking at a steady rate so that ingested calories, carbohydrates and fats can be properly burned. Regular Slimfasting programs will help nourish your pituitary gland and help maintain an active metabolism that will not only take off pounds—but keep them off permanently!

THYROID GLAND— YOUR BODY'S WEIGHT GUARDIAN

Called the "weight guardian" of your body, this biological "clock" can determine whether you are overweight or underweight by the force or weakness of its "ticking."

The thyroid gland is a two-part substance that resembles a butterfly. It rests against the front of your windpipe. It consists of two lobes, one on either side of the Adam's apple, joined at their lower ends by a bridge of glandular tissue across the upper part of the trachea (windpipe).

Under a Slimfasting program, it is able to devote full attention to the secretion of a vital fat-melting hormone known as *thyroxin.* This hormone triggers off the activity or metabolism of the billions of adipose cell tissues.

In particular, the Slimfasting-activated thyroxin hormone helps the body consume oxygen and then burn up accumulated calories, carbohydrates and fats. It is important for the thyroid gland to be adequately nourished. Any imbalance in this "weight guardian" can create disturbances in the quantity of thyroxin being secreted.

Too little thyroxin slows down the burning process and weight is accumulated. Too much thyroxin speeds up the burning process and leads to malnutritious underweight along with rapid breathing and accelerated pulse rate, bulging eyes and nervousness.

Under Slimfasting, the thyroid gland can be "balanced" like a delicate pair of scales so that a sufficient amount of weight-burning thyroxin is secreted and pounds can be healthfully dissolved.

The Everyday Food That
Balances Your Thyroxin Supply

One food contains a substance that becomes nourishment for the thyroid gland. That food is *garlic*. It contains *iodine* in very high concentrations. When you sprinkle a raw salad with garlic powder, or when you chop up a garlic bulb and sprinkle it over a raw salad, you are then sending a rich supply of iodine into your bloodstream to be transported through oxygen carriers right to your thyroid gland. It is this *iodine* that acts as the very source of life to the mainspring of your thyroid clock. Iodine is used by your thyroid to create and balance the supply of thyroxin. Most people get plenty of iodine from table salt, but if you are on a salt-restricted program, you need to obtain it from foods such as seafood and vegetables grown near the ocean.

IODINE STIMULATES WEIGHT-MELTING THYROXIN

Your metabolic process sends iodine into your thyroid gland which then uses it to create thyroxin. Your metabolic process also takes out stored up amino acids from your bloodstream and combines them with the iodine to create a weight-melting reaction. This thyroxin is then transported via your bloodstream to the billions of adipose cell tissues where it helps to break down accumulated weighty substances and propel them out of your system.

How a Slimfasting Garlic Program
Turned Fat into Youthful Muscle

Walter E.D. had more than just an overweight problem. He had developed an unsightly bay window that made him look, feel, and act much older than he really was. No matter how hard he tried, he could not shrink down the bay window. At times, he became so nervous and edgy from food denial that he had to cut into his diet and start stuffing himself. So he welcomed a plan that would give him chewing satisfaction as well as the hope for weight loss.

Walter E.D. followed this easy Slimfasting garlic program:

The first three days of every week (for one month) go on a Slimfasting program consisting of all the raw vegetables that can be eaten with *one* important rule: Each bowl of freshly washed vegetables must be flavored with a chopped or pulverized garlic bulb.

Satisfies Taste, Feels Well Fed, Loses Inches. Almost from the start, Walter E.D. knew this Slimfasting program would give him desired results. He had good taste satisfaction. The garlic-flavored raw vegetables gave him a feeling of being well fed. But most important, *his waistline began to shrink almost daily!* He kept taking in his belt. His clothing had to be taken in, too.

Appetite Is Controlled. The iodine in the garlic combined with the minerals in the vegetables. They were then united by the metabolic process with stored up amino acids to create powerful thyroxin to create a "burning" response so that accumulated calories, carbohydrates, fats could be oxidized and washed out of the system. This gave him a pleasant satisfaction of his appetite. He lost his constant hunger urge. The gnawing compulsion to want to eat was eased. By the end of 17 days, Walter E.D. had actually *lost some 7 inches from his waistline.* He was exhilarated over this simple Slimfasting program using garlic to iodine-nourish his thyroid gland and balance its delicate mechanism so it released a steady hormone supply for weight balance. Soon, Walter E.D. had a slim 32 inch waist. He keeps slim through a twice-a-month Slimfasting program. The first three days of every other week are devoted to raw vegetables sprinkled with much diced or pulverized garlic.

Tip: To help ease or mask the strong odor, eat parsley with your garlic.

How a Slimfasting Seafood Program
Created a Silhouette Figure

Ethel K. had a mischievous thyroid gland. At times, it was sluggish and this led to a thyroxin deficiency and much overweight. At other times, it was hysterically nervous which led to a thunderstorm of thyroxin and a skeleton-like weight loss together with emotional distress. She knew if she could balance the mainsprings of her thyroid gland, she could achieve tranquility as well as a coveted silhouette figure. So she followed a simple and tasty Slimfasting program that consisted solely of seafood together with any desired raw fruits or vegetables. Here was her simple program:

First Day: Fresh fruit for breakfast; fresh fruit with seafood for lunch; fresh fruit with seafood for dinner.

Second Day: Fresh vegetables for breakfast; fresh vegetables with seafood for lunch; fresh vegetables with seafood for dinner.

Third Day: Fresh fruit for breakfast; fresh vegetables with seafood for lunch; fresh fruit with seafood for dinner.

Fourth Day: Fresh fruit juice for breakfast; fresh fruit juice with seafood for lunch; fresh fruit juice with seafood for dinner.

Fifth Day: Fresh vegetable juice for breakfast; fresh vegetable juice with seafood for lunch; fresh vegetable juice with seafood for dinner.

VARIETY IS TASTY SLIMFASTING SPICE OF LIFE

Ethel K. loved this program because of the tasty variety. She could vary the fruits, vegetables, juices and seafood. Each plant food was a different taste thrill. Each type of seafood was another taste adventure. This was a marvelous feast of variety. It gave her the spice of life taste she craved and this made her feel that she was not dieting but enjoying luscious foods.

SLIMFASTING MELTS AWAY POUNDS

The iodine as well as the protein in the seafood combined together with minerals to form the needed thyroxin hormone. The thyroid gland was now *balanced* by the adequate supplies of iodine and thereby helped create a steady "ticking" flow of the weight-melting hormone. Ethel K. lost some 65 pounds with this tasty Slimfasting program. When she reached a slim 118, she could boast she had her coveted silhouette figure. One week every month Ethel K. follows this easy Slimfasting seafood program. The overweight has never come back! She is slim—for life!

Slimfasting Alerts "TSH" Weight-Reducing Action

When you limit intake of food, your metabolism has less "competition" and can now focus full attention on the nutrients of the foods taken in. When you go on a Slimfasting seafood program, *without interference of other foods and elements,* your metabolism is then able to take up the iodine and protein of this seafood and work exclusively with them. Your metabolism takes these nutrients, nourishes the pituitary and thyroid glands and activates them to produce what is known as a "TSH" weight-reducing action.

That is, the iodine-nourished glands promote the formation of a *thyroid stimulating hormone* or TSH which is used to balance body emotions, balance the delicate mainsprings of the glands. This "TSH" action is then able to maintain good metabolism as it works to specifically "burn up" accumulated weighty substances and propel them out of your system.

Under Slimfasting, this TSH action can occur without diversion, without interference, without competition. It is like sending *highly concentrated* iodine to your glands in a potent and *undiluted* form. If you eat seafood with a heavy meal, your digestive system must divide its efforts toward metabolizing all the ingredients. But if you eat seafood plus fruit or vegetables for enzyme activation, then the iodine-mineral-amino acid content is undiluted and can work full force upon your thyroid and other glands. This sends forth a powerful TSH response that can balance your glands and help keep you slim and trim—permanently!

Your glands need to be kept in balanced working order. The hormones or "biological messengers" need to be available in proper supply to create their slimming responses. With regular Slimfasting programs that emphasize gland-feeding nutrients, your body will have hope for taking off weight quickly and permanently!

BASIC BENEFITS

1. Control you "biological clocks" or glands and you can help control your weight.

2. The pituitary gland requires several vitamins and minerals that can help regulate your fat-burning mechanism.

3. The black grape contains gland-nourishing ingredients that can destroy calories. Anna S. lost 48 unwanted pounds under a special Grape Juice Slimfasting program so she looked youthful at the class reunion.

4. Other Slimfasting programs for activation of the pituitary gland are listed for variety and enjoyment as pounds slough off.

5. Nourish your thyroid gland which is your body's weight guardian. Garlic is a powerful source of iodine needed by this gland for its fat-melting power.

6. Walter E.D. lost 7 inches from his waistline under an easy Slimfasting garlic program.

7. Ethel K. tamed her mischievous thyroid gland with a Seafood program that gave her a silhouette figure.

Chapter Sixteen

Youthful Skin, Shaped-Up Body
with Slimfasting

As weight is lost from your body through Slimfasting, other changes are taking place that call for special care of the skin and general condition.

As Slimfasting creates metabolic adjustments so that calories, carbohydrates and fats are "burned" and eliminated, your various body components will undergo other alterations. You will be able to enjoy the rewards of youthful skin and a shaped-up body by following some simple programs. Do these programs *before, during* and *after* your Slimfasting schedule. A combination of these activities with Slimfasting will help adjust your various body systems and a "new you" will emerge.

BETTER POSTURE = BETTER SHAPE

Good posture will give you a good shape. You will also look and feel better. Self-condition yourself to follow these rules for better posture:

STANDING. Stand erect with you head high, chin in, shoulders back, chest up, abdomen flat, hips down, knees straight, feet parallel, weight well balanced. *Avoid* a strained, exaggerated position. *Remember:* a drooping head, rounded shoulders, hollow chest and sagging abdomen are contrary to good posture and make you look older. So stand properly and look slimmer.

WALKING. Carry your body as when standing. Walk freely, feet parallel and close together. Hold yourself tall but not taut, and breathe deeply lifting your chest walls for full expansion. Let your arms hang loosely at your sides. You will soon enjoy the feeling of this new freedom in walking.

SITTING. Sit well back in your chair with the end of your spine touching the back of your chair and your body erect but not stiff. Place your feet directly in front of you so that you are comfortable. If you sit many hours a day at your work be sure to use a chair that supports your body properly. Avoid a slouching position that throws your body off balance.

SLEEPING. Use a firm mattress to keep your body in good position while you are at rest. The box or innerspring type that supports all parts of your body equally is particularly good. You can avoid a backache by putting firm support beneath an uncomfortable and otherwise sagging mattress.

CHECKING-UP. Check-up on yourself regularly by standing against a wall. Head, shoulders, buttocks, calves and heels should all touch, with the hollow of your back just deep enough for your fingers. Facing the wall your chest should touch first.

EASY FITNESS WHILE SLIMFASTING

Keep your body active while you Slimfast. This helps improve your circulatory-metabolic processes and there is an increased "burning" of accumulated weighty substances. Here are some suggestions for easy fitness while Slimfasting:

WALKING. This is an excellent over-all body conditioner during Slimfasting. Decide to walk every time you do not absolutely have to ride. Step along briskly, breathe deeply. Begin your walking with about half a mile daily and gradually increase it up to two or three miles per day. Take friends or family along.

SPORTS. You need not be an expert to enjoy and benefit from such activities as swimming, golf, dancing, bowling, Ping-Pong, tennis, badminton. Bicycling is also healthful. You can pedal vigorously until your muscles have had enough. Then you can relax and coast until your muscles are ready for more. Bicycling, like brisk walking, speeds the flow of blood back to the heart. This improves your health during Slimfasting.

CLIMBING-STRETCHING. Take the stairs at every opportunity, instead of an elevator or escalator. Stretch, too, especially when your muscles feel tense. The simple act of stretching is a fine exercise for anyone who must sit at a desk or table for long hours in a fixed position.

IN-BED EXERCISE. Pretend you are a rubber band. Raise both arms over your head and stretch both your hands and feet away from your middle, stretching and reaching as far as you possibly can. Relax and collapse just like a rubber band. Stretch, relax, collapse—that's the technique. Start doing it five times each morning before you get out of bed, increasing each day by one until you have reached at least twenty. You'll feel so alive you'll leap out of bed like a gazelle.

THE WALL EXERCISE. Stand against a wall, with your heels about four inches away from the base of the wall. Now bend your knees, slowly, all the way down while keeping the small of your back pressed tight to the wall and your head touching the wall. This takes practice and you should try to work up to ten times. Gradually, of course. This exercise will help tighten stomach muscles during Slimfasting, remind you to keep your buttocks flat and help give you a good carriage.

THE STRETCH EXERCISE. Stand with your feet about 18 inches apart and stretch your arms straight out to the side. Now bend sideways, reaching down with your left hand to your left ankle and up toward the ceiling with your right hand. Keep your head turned to the right. Reverse procedure, reaching for your right ankle and stretching left hand toward ceiling. This time, keep head turned left. Start by doing five each day and work up to at least twenty. This exercise stretches every muscle in your body during Slimfasting and you'll feel loose-limbed and agile.

YOUTHFUL SKIN AND HEALTHY HAIR WITH SLIMFASTING

As toxins and wastes are cast out of your body during Slimfasting, an internal purification process occurs. You will be rewarded with a more youthful skin and better hair texture when your internal viscera are cleansed. Because there is going to be a great deal of water loss as wastes are transported out of your eliminative channels, you should plan to consume as many liquids as is comfortable. This helps to rehydrate your system, moisturize your skin and scalp cells and guard against external aging reactions.

Here is an assortment of different all-natural home remedies to help keep your skin youthful and your hair healthy during Slimfasting:

SOAP-FREE CLEANSER. Any polyunsaturated oil (olive oil, peanut oil, safflower oil, corn oil) may be used as a soap-free skin cleanser. Dip fingertips in the oil and massage upward and in a circular motion all over your face. Then tissue off. Helps lubricate your skin and does not upset the acid-alkaline balance as may occur with soaps.

WRINKLED EYELIDS. Bathe wrinkled and tired eyes in a warm salt solution of 1/2 teaspoon of salt to a pint of water.

PUFFED EYES. Apply pads wrung out of a solution of a pint of comfortably hot water and 1 teaspoon of salt. Lie back and relax while this remedy does its soothing work.

DULL, LIFELESS HAIR. Make it glossy and shiny with this dry shampoo: 1 ounce of powdered orris root (from herbal pharmacies) with 1/2 pound of salt. Rub well into your scalp, then brush out briskly.

TIGHT SCALP. Stimulate your scalp and get rid of flakiness (a symptom of internal cleansing during Slimfasting) with a pack made of 1 cup of salt and 5 tablespoons water. Rub this paste into your scalp, let it remain for 5 minutes, then remove by brisk rubbing and a shampoo.

RED, WRINKLED HANDS. Soak for 5 minutes in a basin of warm water to which 3 tablespoons of salt have been added.

TIRED, ACHING FEET. Soak in a warm bath to which a generous handful of salt has been added. If especially sore, soak alternately in a hot salt brine. Massage gently with moistened salt to remove dry skin, rinse in cool water and dry thoroughly. Dust with talcum or foot powder.

AGING SKIN. Try a stimulating facial. Mix equal portions of salt and olive oil and gently massage face and throat with long, upward strokes. Let the mixture remain for 5 minutes, then remove with facial tissues. Wash face with mild soap and water.

OVERALL FATIGUE. How to overcome the fatigued-tired feeling often experienced with slimming. Here's a remedy used by a formerly overweight active mother and clubwoman, Judith P. She would toss one cup of salt into a tub of warm water, then relax in the briny depths for 30 minutes. Judith P. would emerge with renewed vitality and energy. Slimfasting never tired her, because of this simple remedy.

COMPLEXION PROBLEMS. Whether sallow, dull or lifeless, you can make yourself glow during Slimfasting with either of these two facial masks which draw out the impurities sent to your skin surface during weight loss. They also help refine your complexion and make you glow all over:

- Lightly beat an egg white. Mix in 1 tablespoon of mayonnaise and 1 tablespoon of lemon juice. Spread on face and neck and allow to dry. Rinse with warm water.

- Mix 1 egg white and 1/2 cup lemon juice with sufficient dry oatmeal to make a paste. Apply to face and neck and allow to dry. Rinse with warm water.

CHAPPED HANDS. Rub your hands with lemon juice to help restore the natural acid mantle of the skin which is often removed as wastes are washed out of your system during this Slimfasting program. Lemon juice helps soothe hands (and skin, in general) and keep you looking youthful as pounds slough off.

GENERAL SKIN CARE. You'll need to re-establish the delicate acid-alkaline balance of your skin during Slimfasting. Do it easily with this remedy: Beat two egg yolks in a cold bowl. Slowly, as you beat, add one cup of corn oil. Now add just enough oatmeal or cornstarch until you have a paste that can be spread. Also add one tablespoon of apple cider vinegar. Now spread all over your face. Let it remain for 30 to 45 minutes or longer. Then splash off with contrasting warm and cold water. This helps acidify your skin so it is youthful and soft to appearance and touch.

DRY BODY SKIN. Rub yourself all over with ordinary body oil. Now sit in a steamy tub. Luxuriate for 30 to 45 minutes. The steam will open your pores, remove impurities and permit the oil to enter. This total body lubrication helps keep your skin smooth. It protects against dry skin, the bane of many reducing programs.

WRINKLE-ERASER. Although she lost some 74 pounds and at least 10 inches, Marion L.L. has a youthful wrinkle-free skin. Her secret is this 30 minute facial tightener: Peel out the still-moist membrane or white lining of an egg shell after you prepare eggs. Apply this still-moist membranous white lining all over your face. It is pure protein, that tends to adhere to creases, furrows, wrinkles. Let it remain for 30 minutes. Then splash off with cool water. Pat dry. Marion L.L. does this every few days. She has a remarkably smooth and wrinkle-free skin. No matter how much weight she loses, her skin remains firm, smooth and baby-clear, thanks to this simple remedy.

CROW'S FEET. As weight is lost out of your body, the bony sockets of the eyes may look hollow. To avoid crow's feet setting in, try this easy remedy: Hold an icy wet washcloth against your closed eyes for 5 minutes. Then dry gently. This helps tighten up the skin and guard against crow's feet.

SKIN DRYNESS. Ordinary Vaseline or petroleum jelly is a helpful lubricant, especially around the eyes or any areas where there are fine lines. Just rub a thin film in and around the area. Do this gently. If possible, let it remain for several hours or throughout the day. It moisturizes your skin, keeps it looking supple, smooth, soft during Slimfasting and afterwards, too.

DRY HAIR. Dip fingertips into corn oil or baby oil. Rub thoroughly into your scalp. Then brush. In no time at all, your hair is healthy and shining.

BODY SKIN. Give yourself a total body "facial" by adding one cup of cornstarch, 1/2 cup of milk, 1/2 cup of mineral oil to a warm tub. Now immerse yourself. Luxuriate up to 45 minutes. The warm water will steam open your pores to enable your Slimfasting-released toxic wastes to make a swift exit. The blend of the ingredients helps moisturize cells beneath the skin surface, "plumps" up tissues, guards against wrinkling and aging. It's the "fun" way to relax your way to a youthful skin while Slimfasting.

TWO-CENT WRINKLE-FREE SECRET. Mary Ann O'G. needed to lose much of her accumulated overweight. She saw others develop wrinkled skin, deep, unsightly folds after having lost weight. To guard against this age threat, Mary Ann O'G. used what she called a "2¢ wrinkle-free secret" remedy. For most of the day and even overnight, Mary Ann O'G. would put a thin film of oil on her face, throat and other visible sections that would ordinarily be prone to wrinkling. She preferred *baby oil* because it was made from only the purest ingredients under the most stringent laboratory conditions. She said it cost her only 2¢ per application. Yet, it kept her skin remarkably free from wrinkling. Even after she lost some 40 pounds, her skin was firm, glowing, as if she had roses in her cheeks. *Little-Known Benefit:* Baby oil is important in helping to replace moisture and body oils that diminish and often dry up during weight loss. Baby oil protects the skin against the loss of its all-important elasticity. *Baby oil prevents skin drought* during weight loss. It's the easy, low-cost way to keep your skin in the "prime of life" during Slimfasting. All this for only 2¢ per application!

BLEMISHES. These often are symptomatic of the body's readjustment during Slimfasting. To ease, just apply buttermilk over affected area. Then splash off with tingling cool water. Helps neutralize acid waste accumulation, tightens the pores and makes your skin look smoother.

IRRITATING ITCH. Often weight loss may make the skin feel itchy or "crawly." It is a symptomatic reaction to the biological changes in your body. To ease, just baby yourself in two easy ways: (1) Before a bath, rub the itching area with a fine film of baby oil. Let it soak in for 30 to 45 minutes before immersing yourself in a tepid bath. Then use a gentle washcloth to wash yourself. (2) After the bath, towel dry yourself gently and now dust your itching parts with baby powder. This helps ease the itch and make you feel good all over.

Slimfasting is a natural and easy way to lose stubborn pounds and inches from your body while you rejuvenate your skin and shape-up your body. Total youthfulness is a possible dream when you follow the natural programs as outlined above.

IN REVIEW

1. Readjust to your new slim weight with better posture.
2. Keep yourself fit with the outlined no-fuss, no-effort exercises.

3. Judith P. overcame fatigue during weight loss with a simple salt water tub bath. Just 30 minutes gave her zest and pep.

4. Protect yourself against wrinkles and scalp disorders with the outlined all-natural programs.

5. Marion L.L. has a youthful wrinkle-free skin even after losing 74 pounds and 10 inches. She uses the white lining of an egg shell for wrinkle prevention.

6. Mary Ann O'G. uses a 2¢ baby oil application and is rewarded with a youthful peaches-and-cream skin after losing 40 pounds.

Chapter Seventeen

How to Use Slimfasting

to Improve Your Health

Easy-to-follow Slimfasting programs can do more than help take off stubborn pounds and unsightly inches. These programs can improve your basic health and start you on the road to recuperation from such ailments as heart distress, hardening of the arteries, diabetes, digestive disorders, and many other disorders. For problems with arteriosclerosis, diabetes, digestive disorders, and so on, you should be guided by your doctor's advice. Cooperate with him by further improving your nutritional practices so you enable your body to invigorate from within to boost better health. Slimfasting offers a double-barrelled benefit by slimming you down and also improving your basic health.

SLIMFASTING WILL HELP
ADD YEARS TO YOUR LIFE

As pounds and inches roll off through Slimfasting, you will be able to add years to your life. Illness is less likely to afflict the normal weight person. Putting it simply, *the slimmer the belt line, the longer the life line.* (See Figure 17-1.)

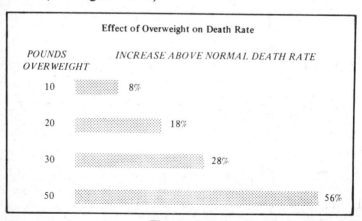

Figure 17-1

SLIMFASTING FOR A LONGER HEART LINE

Lengthen your heart line through a simple Slimfasting program that controls the intake of fat and calories. One such program was followed by the meat-loving Roger C. who had an insatiable urge for heavy, fatty casseroles and stews. He was a hard-driving executive, frequently going on sales trips during which he would eat heavily in restaurants, disregarding his expanding waistline and his heavy breathing. Roger C. loved the taste of fatty meats too much to want to give them up, even when his doctor told him that it was a matter of life and death!

HEAVY WEIGHT, HEAVY BREATHING, RAPID HEARTBEAT

Roger C. carried around 52 extra pounds; he wheezed and sputtered and gasped when he walked up a few steps and succumbed to heavy breathing; his heart pounded at a furious rate upon the least bit of physical and/or emotional exertion. When he began to experience dizzy spells and a loss of balance, his doctor demanded that Roger do something. Yet, he was insistent upon not giving up his love for heavy foods. With this in mind, he decided to follow a Slimfasting program.

Slimfasting for Healthier Heart

Here is the tasty "fat-satisfying" Slimfasting program followed by Roger C. that lengthened his life and heart line:

1. Daily, eat very lean chicken and turkey. (Poultry fat is evenly distributed between hard and soft fat ratios.)

2. Enjoy a meat loaf that is made with diced chicken or turkey and just a small amount of beef chuck to give it a disguised flavor satisfaction.

3, Increase intake of fish that is prepared with vegetable oil.

4. Replace butter with polyunsaturated margarine. This cholesterol or animal fat-free product gives all the taste satisfaction of fat but is comparatively heart-healthy.

5. Enjoy a wide variety of dairy products made from skim milk. The taste is just about the same but it is weight-losing and heart-healthy.

6. *Basic Slimfasting Program:* Roger C. ate *more frequent smaller meals* instead of a few larger ones. *Benefit:* This Slimfasting program enables your digestive organs better assimilation power than if you suddenly eat a huge meal.

Smaller meals are better metabolized and there is less build-up time in the adipose cell tissues and consequently less weight gain. It is also much more soothing to the heart.

7. For one meal, Roger C. drank two cups of broth, consomme or bouillon. *Benefit:* This low-calorie Slimfasting program introduced much liquid into his digestive system so that accumulated wastes and toxins could then be washed out of the body.

8. Favorite stews, casseroles could be enjoyed if made largely with vegetables, if polyunsaturated cooking oils were used, if chicken and turkey were blended in with smaller portions of meats. This would offer the satisfaction Roger C. needed for his "fat love" but would also be much lower in calories as well as saturated fat.

9. Eating time was scheduled. This prevented habitual overeating and gulping down of large amounts of foods. Roger C. was told to do nothing but eat at the smaller meals. He was to focus full attention upon the food (no matter how small, even if only a beverage) that he was consuming. This would give him good appetite-satisfaction.

10. Finally, he devoted two days per week to a raw juice fast; one day could be raw fruit juice. The other day could be raw vegetable juice.

RESULTS? WEIGHT EVAPORATES, BREATHING STABILIZES, HEARTBEAT CALMS

Roger C. weighed himself daily under this program and was delighted to see the pounds actually "evaporate" as he began to slim down. Soon, his breathing was stabilized and his heartbeat was calm. But more important to Roger C., this Slimfasting program lets him enjoy his favorite fatty foods (disguised as polyunsaturated vegetable fats) so he does not feel he is dieting! After three months, at a slim 135 pounds, Roger C. now has a new lease on his heart line!

HOW TO "SLIMFAST-SCRUB" YOUR ARTERIES

Arteriosclerosis or "hardening of the arteries" is frequently the result of a lifetime of heavy, fatty food intake. Many folks want to enjoy the taste of fat while they are on an "artery-washing" program. Slimfasting can help scrub the cholesterol and other fatty deposits from your arteries so that you will be naturally protected against the risk of arteriosclerosis.

Slimfasting on Plant Foods for
Cholesterol-Control

Because cholesterol is found solely in foods of animal origin, you will help control buildup of this fatty substance by following a Slimfasting program of a wide variety of any desired plant foods. Here is one tasty program:

First Day: Ease into your Slimfasting by devoting the entire day to small meals of slightly steamed or simmered vegetables. You may enjoy slices of freshly baked eggplant seasoned with herbs and spices; try a platter of steamed cabbage, mushrooms, split peas. A baked potato with a flavoring of parsley and garlic powder is healthful. Select three to four small meals that are spaced out during the day, consisting of any desired seasonal vegetables.

Second Day: Devote entirely to fresh raw fruits in a variety of salads and platters. Enjoy apples, bananas, seasonal berries, various melons, platters of grapes, an assortment of seasonal citrus fruits. Again, schedule four small meals which are devoted to different assortments of raw fruits.

Third Day: Liquefy your system with an all-day raw vegetable juice fast. Select any desired juice-bearing vegetables such as tomatoes, lettuce, celery, carrots, beets and then juice them and enjoy them either singly or in a variety of different combinations. You may schedule juice intakes as if they were regular meals if you feel that will give you a feeling of satisfaction.

Fourth Day: At this time, your digestive system is ready to be "energized" and "alerted" to scrub away the accumulated debris that is cholesterol from your arteries. After three days of *total plant food intake,* the hardened deposits have become softened. They can be more easily dissolved and sloughed off. Raw fruit juices will provide the energy and power to create this process. Devote the entire day to raw fruit juices. Your digestive system will use the enzymes and vitamins from raw fruit juices to help alert the metabolism so that excess cholesterol in the arteries can be "burned up." Select a variety of different favorite fruits such as apples, oranges, pears, grapefruits, berries; juice them either singly or in tasty combinations. Then drink either at scheduled times or just freely throughout the day. You'll feel your viscera (internal organs) being scrubbed clean as the cholesterol deposits are loosened and then washed out of your body.

Fifth Day: You are now going to break your fast so do it gently, do it easily and slowly. Begin with this meal pattern: *Breakfast:* Applesauce flavored with honey; bowl of all-natural cereal or bran with skim milk and sun-dried raisins; whole grain toast with a dab of margarine; herb tea. *Luncheon:* Steamed brown rice with margarine;

baked eggplant with mushrooms; cup vegetable broth; herb tea. *Dinner:* Baked potato with dab of oil; steamed squash with herbal flavorings; lettuce-tomato salad; whole grain bread; herb tea.

Sixth Day: Now you slowly ease into a soft boiled egg (limit to three weekly) for breakfast with seasonal fruits; for luncheon, enjoy a grilled cheese-tomato sandwich and seasonal fruits; for dinner, try lean fish with lemon slices, slightly steamed vegetables, whole grain bread, herb tea.

Afterwards: Emphasize intake of *lean* meats with turkey and chicken as the most preferred. Limit eggs to three weekly. Dairy products should be made of skimmed milk. Every single meal MUST have either a large fruit or vegetable salad. This is needed to provide your system with enzymes. Enzymes are protein-like substances in raw fruits and vegetables that help boost body metabolism to scrub away cholesterol. Often, the body's own enzyme supply may be weak, hence the need for a daily supply from raw plant foods. Just as you fortify your protein store with protein foods, boost your enzyme levels with enzyme foods.

Slimfasting Benefits: This simple 6-day program is aimed at helping your metabolic process adjust itself so that accumulated wastes and toxins can then be washed out of your system. Your arteries can be scrubbed and transformed into youthful "branches" in the "tree" of your body, giving you a healthy cholesterol-controlled lifeline for longer years and better health.

SLIMFASTING FOR RELIEF OF DIABETES

An overworked glandular-metabolic system may often become "exhausted" so that some weakening or malfunctioning may be the consequence. One such condition is that of diabetes, which is traced to a weakness of the pancreatic gland in secreting enough insulin. Insulin is needed to break down sugar and other carbohydrates into more simple sugars. Insulin also breaks down glucose (simple sugar) into carbon dioxide and water. It helps in the storage of glycogen (a starch) in the liver for use whenever needed.

An overworked pancreas will become exhausted so that it secretes less insulin and this may cause a buildup of sugar in the system and thereby create a condition known as diabetes.

SLIMFASTING HELPS PANCREAS REGENERATE

A simple Slimfasting program is helpful in giving the glandular-metabolic system, especially the pancreas (large, long organ situated behind the lower portion of the stomach) a much-needed recuperative process that will strengthen its function. Slimfasting helps the pancreas regenerate so that it can then secrete more supplies of needed insulin for sugar metabolism.

SLIMFASTING ALERTS BETTER INSULIN PRODUCTION

Adelle A.R. was over 40 and also overweight. She had constant thirst, was frequently "edgy" and also was told she was on the verge of serious diabetes. Adelle A.R. wanted to use a natural approach that would perform two basic benefits: first, take off the 33 unwanted pounds and many inches; second, correct her glandular-metabolic "clocks" so that there would be no risk of diabetes. On the advice of a friend, she followed an easy Slimfasting program:

First Day of Fruit: She could eat all she wanted of these fruits (raw) for the entire day: apples, apricots, bananas, blackberries, blueberries, cantaloupe, cherries, figs, grapes, grapefruits, oranges, peaches, pears, pineapples, plums, prunes, raspberries, strawberries, watermelon. *Note:* These should be fresh; but if frozen or canned, they must be *without* sugar.

Sceond Day of Vegetables. Adelle A.R. could eat all she wanted of these vegetables (either raw, or if cooked, steamed slightly to make palatable but NOT prepared with salt or vinegar) for the entire day: asparagus, cucumbers, peppers, broccoli, Brussels sprouts, cabbage, cauliflower, celery, eggplant, greens, lettuce, mushrooms, okra, radishes, stringbeans, tomatoes. *Note:* These should be fresh; but if frozen or canned, they must be *without* sugar.

Third Day of Juices. Adelle A.R. could drink all she wanted of fresh fruit or vegetable juices. For better metabolism, she would *not* combine them. Instead, she would space an hour or more between juices if she wanted to drink fruit and then vegetable elixirs.

Fourth Day to Ease out of Fast: She could now eat whole grain cereals, soft boiled eggs, lean meat and low-fat fish. She would do this slowly to ease out of her fast.

HORMONES BECOME HEALTHY, ABUNDANT

Adelle A.R. followed this Slimfasting program the first three days of every week. The rest of the week, she made it a rule to AVOID refined sugar in any form, whether from the sugar bowl or in cooked foods. She also selected foods that were both low calorie and low carbohydrate (but high in protein). These gave her a balanced eating program. (*Note:* Charts listing these foods are found in this book.) As a result, Adelle A.R. lost the 33 unwanted pounds and many inches. She was overjoyed at the way her scale reading kept going down and down. And more joyful was the news that her pancreas had regenerated itself and a healthy supply of abundant insulin erased the risk of diabetes.

Now, Adelle A.R. follows this easy *First Three Days Of Each Week Slimfasting* program. It keeps her slim. It protects her against the threat of diabetes.

Benefits: When Adelle A.R. followed the preceding program, she restricted the consumption of calories and carbohydrates. This gave her pancreas a much needed respite. The gland could now work at a healthy pace. In particular, when the metabolic system is spared being overloaded with carbohydrates and sugars, the pancreas can then *balance* a *steady* supply of needed insulin. This protects against a condition known as "insulin antagonism" which occurs through overeating. In this condition, a weakened insulin supply causes the formation of a substance known as *synalbumin* in the blood cells; this substance blocks the full use of insulin. To avoid formation of *synalbumin,* a Slimfasting program helps to prevent pancreatic overloading. This gland can then devote full attention to secretion of insulin to work upon the reduced amount of calories and carbohydrates. This helps create better "burning" and healthy weight loss. Specifically, *Slimfasting helps neutralize the pressure on the pancreas.* This creates a better balanced flow of insulin and a natural protection against diabetes.

REJUVENATE YOUR DIGESTIVE SYSTEM WITH SLIMFASTING

You can help ease and erase the consequences of improper eating and digestive disturbance with regular Slimfasting. Basically, a Slimfasting program should neutralize acid, soothe digestive function, be comfortable, supply needed bulk. While the emphasis here is on *natural* and nonprocessed foods, it is more important to plan to be good to your digestive system, to pamper it so it will reward you with comfort and pleasure.

Basic Slimfasting Program

1. If overweight, cut your food portions in half.
2. Eliminate all alcoholic beverages, volatile spices such as salt, pepper, vinegar. Do not use these in any form. Instead, flavor with more natural herbs.
3. Foods should NOT be fried. This causes an excessive outpouring of pancreatic and gastic juices which will give you

a bloated reaction and sour taste. Eliminate fried foods in all forms.

4. If you have stomach upset or recurring disorders, then go on a Slimfasting program that begins with two days of liquids only. On the third day, you may have vegetable broths, well-broiled meat. You slowly increase with thoroughly chewed fruits or vegetables and skim milk products.

5. Increase intake of fish (baked, broiled, boiled but NEVER fried) that is mashed or cut into tiny pieces that are easy to chew and easy to swallow.

6. All fruits and vegetables should have skin, pits and roughage removed for better digestion.

7. To guard against constipation or diverticulosis (development of small pouches along the colon where food may lodge and cause irritation) increase intake of bran. Use whole, non-processed bran sprinkled over a mashed fruit or vegetable dish, or combine with skim milk yogurt or add to a stew or casserole. Bran helps speed up transit time of bulk in the system and guards against retention which causes digestive unrest.

8. Plan a Slimfasting program of frequent small feedings. This is soothing to your digestive system.

9. Foods to be eliminated are smoked meats, spiced foods, rich buttery foods, fried foods, egg and milk fillings such as custards, anything made with refined sugar, anything made with salt, pepper, vinegar or chemical preservatives.

10. Devote one day a week to a total raw fruit juice fast.

11. Devote one day a week to a total raw vegetable juice fast.

12. For persistent inflammation, devote 24 to 48 hours to total fasting. The only intake consists of water.

With these Slimfasting programs, you should be able to rebuild your digestive system, lose weight, melt away inches, cleanse your internal organism so that you will help adjust your metabolism for better health.

You may vary your Slimfasting programs, unless you need one for a specific condition. Otherwise, try one Slimfasting program for one week, then go to another one. This creates variety and helps give your body all types of healing responses. You will also be losing unwanted weight. This, in itself, is your key to better health, longer life and total rejuvenation!

HIGHLIGHTS

1. Live longer and better and correct health problems with regular Slimfasting.

2. Roger C. went on a Slimfasting program that caused weight loss, improved the health of his heart and gave him a longer lifeline.

3. You can "Slimfast-Scrub" cholesterol from your arteries and guard against arteriorsclerosis.

4. Adelle A.R. used a Slimfasting program that protected her against diabetes while taking off unwanted pounds and inches.

5. Rebuild-rejuvenate your digestive system with easy-to-follow Slimfasting.

Chapter Eighteen

65 Slimfasting Hints and Tips
for Fast Weight Loss

"BIG POUNDS FROM LITTLE OUNCES GROW"

Pounds and inches accumulate from daily nibblings, little errors that tend to cause fat accumulation. You can follow easy Slimfasting hints and tips in daily living to help keep off those unwanted pounds. Here is an assortment of these suggestions that you can follow in your daily eating or Slimfasting programs:

1. Spread a *thin* topping. If your Slimfasting program suggests a bread topping, do it very thinly. A very thin spread will give you taste but with far fewer calories.

2. For a good digestive stimulus, try freshly washed lettuce. Whenever you want to alert your sluggish digestion, nibble on washed lettuce that can be flavored with parsley or garlic or onion powder or other soothing herbs.

3. You may have the urge to nibble between meals or during a Slimfasting program. If so, try such low-calorie foods as: carrot sticks, celery nuggets, raw mushroom caps, cauliflower buds. They satisfy the eating urge but are very low in calories. Eat in moderation, if on a liquid program.

4. Soothe your taste buds and tongue papillae with a lukewarm mouth wash. Add a half teaspoon of baking soda, swirl around and then rinse. You'll find your appetite easing. Also, you'll feel refreshed all over. Helps wash out accumulated wastes, too.

5. Any solid foods eaten during a Slimfasting program should be cut in small pieces. This gives you more chewing satisfaction, avoids gulping and makes you feel "filled up" with less food.

6. Concentrate on each bite and mouthful of food (or sip of liquid) you consume. This will also offer great satisfaction with smaller amounts.

7. Drink as much water throughout the day as is comfortably possible. Helps take the edge off your appetite and also helps wash out toxic wastes from your fasting system.

8.   If you anticipate a weekend that will call for much eating, prepare for it in advance. Go on a total fast one or two days during the week or afterwards, consuming only water or low-calorie celery or carrot juice. This "compensates" for the added calories you took in during your feast.

9.   Replace heavy butter with cholesterol-free margarine or polyunsaturated oils. TIP: Scramble eggs with skim milk instead of butter or margarine for very low calorie count.

10.   Self-test yourself daily to guard against sneaking inches and pounds. Example: mark your belt to a desired girth and use a hook in that hole; daily, see if the belt gets too tight since that means more pounds and inches. Try not to go out of that "Slimfasting hole" in your belt.

11.   When flavoring your Slimfasting foods, use low calorie ingredients. Example, use ordinary tomato juice or puree as a sauce or topping. Low-calorie broths and powders are also good.

12.   Mash some apples and use as a topping for rye wafers or on a slice of skim milk cheese for a little low-calorie treat.

13.   If you must snack, try chestnuts! An average hot-roasted chestnut offers you a low 4 or 5 calories. Also offers taste-satisfaction.

14.   Another low-calorie snack is ordinary popcorn (but don't use butter or margarine or salt; only herbs and spices). Eat a few of them. Wash down with water.

15.   You'll resist the temptation to snack by not having any high calorie or high fat foods in your house. Keep them away. Keep away from them, too! This goes for cookies, candies, cakes, etc.

16.   If your Slimfasting program includes meats or fish, be sure to trim off all visible fats *before* eating. DO NOT leave the fat on your plate. Discard it. Less tempting if it cannot be seen.

17.   Here's how to enjoy a low-fat natural beef gravy for a topping. Drop a few ice cubes into a bowl of this gravy. Soon, you'll see fat rising to the bowl top. It becomes solid. Remove and discard with a spoon. You'll then have tasty, high-protein but low-fat beef gravy.

18.   Here's how to enjoy low-fat soup if it's made of meat stock: float a lettuce leaf on top for a few moments. Much of the fat tends to stick to this leaf. Remove the leaf and discard.

19.   Contrast allowable vegetables to give you better eye appeal. Different colors tossed together make a rainbow that is visually pleasing, digestively and metabolically satisfying.

20.   If your Slimfasting program lists cooked foods, then use broiling, baking, boiling or roasting. This makes the foods more digestible. An added benefit is that these methods cause the fat to settle upon and around the meat so you can skim off much of it.

21.   Put exciting taste in any food with flavorings of herbs and spices. Select any of your favorites and use according to taste. Even a glass of tomato juice is sparkled up with a sprinkle of parsley.

22.   Indulge yourself in lots of low-calorie garnishes for any meals. Enjoy shredded carrots, cucumber slices, watercress, parsley. They make a flavorful accompaniment to any meal. They take monotony out of any food.

23.   Pep up any raw vegetable salad with a sprinkle of fresh lemon or lime juice. You may also use a bit of apple cider vinegar and oil with desired herbs for a low-calorie dressing.

24.   If Slimfasting suggests dairy products, be sure they are made of skim milk. The label will tell you so. Use skim milk products for cooking, too.

25.   If on a raw fruit or vegetable fast, make each item look like a meal with the use of various gadgets. You can shred, grate, chop, slice, make myriads of designs so that a carrot can look different each time it is eaten!

26.   Here's how to make a delicious *Slimfasting Tonic,* as used by a busy housewife who wanted to take the edge off her appetite. Dora MacA. wanted a high-protein, low-calorie and appetite-pleasing "in-a-flash" tonic. This is what she used when she went on any Slimfasting program that made her feel occasional hunger: Combine 1 glass of skim milk, 1 tablespoon of Postum, 1/2 teaspoon honey, 1 egg white. Beat until thick and frothy. Sip slowly. *Benefit:* Your resting metabolic system can take the pure and complete protein of the egg white, use the high vitamin-mineral content of the skim milk and propel these nutrients towards the billions of your body cells to nourish them as they are being fat-scrubbed. Egg white contains a complete protein. Skim milk contains an incomplete protein, so combine with egg white for better balance. There is also a feeling of appetite satisfaction as the egg white uses the minerals of the skim milk to coat the digestive organ and soothe its contractions. Dora MacA. uses this *Slimfasting Tonic* daily. She feels great as pounds and inches melt away.

27.   Get into the good habit of serving yourself *smaller* portions. *Never* overstuff yourself. Visually, a smaller portion on a smaller plate should offer you good emotional satisfaction.

28.   Whenever you feel filled up, discard or store the leftover food. Do not delay. Do not let it sit on your plate. This is too tempting. *Out of sight—out of appetite!*

29.   If you eat alone, then focus all attention upon your food. DO NOT watch television or read while eating. This does not give you full satisfaction, and the divided attention tends to make you overeat. When you eat—do just that: *eat!*

30.   When eating with others, DO NOT talk with food in your mouth. First chew, swallow your food. Put down utensils before talking. Be aware of the difference between talking and eating. DO NOT combine both activities.

31.   Foods should be chewed, savored, swallowed leisurely. DO NOT wash down foods with liquids. If you are on a liquid fast, then sip, savor and swallow slowly. Make the most out of every morsel or drop for better satisfaction.

32.   Concentrate on the taste, texture and temperature of whatever you are eating or drinking. Tell yourself how sweet, tangy, tart, smooth, rough, hot, or cold it is. This gives you greater enjoyment, even for very small quantities.

33.   Be seated when you eat or drink. You'll find you're more satisfied when seated. This was discovered by Neal O'P. He found that on any Slimfasting program, he could eat-enjoy and satisfy himself with less, if he *sat down,* even for a glass of a juice. But when Neal O'P. stood up, he found he wanted to eat more. When he made this simple adjustment of sitting down for any intake of food or liquid, Neal O'P. lost his unwanted pounds and inches and felt totally satisfied with smaller amounts. Sitting helps you become aware of your behavior. Standing tempts you to unconsciously keep on eating and eating.

34.   To avoid temptation, try the *Slimfasting law of compensation:* Instead of a piece of cake, try a scoop of cottage cheese. Instead of a high calorie malted, try a low-calorie herb tea or vegetable juice. Give in to oral satisfaction with a substitute food; this compensates and satisfies. If you cannot resist temptation, again try the Slimfasting law of compensation but *in reverse:* eat your icing-topped cupcake, eat your chocolate eclair, and then compensate by skipping a meal or going on a one-day Slimfasting juice program. This will balance your caloric intake and permit your metabolism to burn up accumulated fats. But before you indulge in a "no no" food, plan ahead. Tell yourself that you can eat a large wedge of apple pie a la mode but ONLY if you will compensate by skipping one meal the next day. Do not cheat on your promise to yourself! You'll only be fooling yourself—not the scale!

35.   When dining at a friend's home, if your hostess says, "This is my very special apple pie so can't you make an exception just this once?" you can try this Slimfasting trick: ask for a small portion, eat a very small amount of it and leave the rest on your plate. Otherwise, tell your host or hostess *in advance,* when you accept the dinner invitation, that you are Slimfasting and must adhere to the schedule.

36.   For some folks, losing weight is easier with a companion or

a group. Get together with other overweights and Slimfast in groups. It may give you the emotional support you need.

37. To help combat early morning constipation, try this Slimfasting suggestion: the night before, soak six prunes in a glass of water or in a glass of orange or grapefruit juice. In the morning, drink this beverage. Eat the pitted prunes. It helps create regularity whether or not you are on Slimfasting.

38. Once you have selected your Slimfasting program, make no changes unless absolutely necessary. Any change may disrupt the reflex response and your appetite goes awry. Keep a schedule. Avoid variations for Slimfasting success.

39. Eat small amounts of raw vegetables *before* a protein meal because the natural carbohydrates stimulate the pancreas to secrete more sugar-burning insulin. Raw vegetable carbohydrates also tend to create a metabolic reaction whereby fat is "pulled out" of the fat depots in your body and washed out of the system. Eating raw vegetables *before* a protein meal sets off this chain reaction. It is the easy and effortless way to wash fat out of your body.

40. If you are faced with the temptation to overeat, pause and reflect. Visualize a very fat, corpulent person. Mentally "hear" jeers and laughter at a roly-poly. Listen to the taunts of "Hey, fatty," or "Hi, big tub of lard," or "Hey, fat slob." This helps control your appetite since you won't want to be so insulted.

41. During a Slimfasting program, make a ritual out of each and every course. Set a table as if for a feast. Use your best table settings. Make a little bit of food or drink go a long way!

42. If your Slimfasting program calls for a few items, then try to put them all on one plate. For example: sliced chicken, fresh fruit slices, sliced cucumbers-peppers-carrots can all go on one sectioned plate. It makes it appear like a large meal if served on one plate instead of a few of them.

43. And always use a smaller plate so that the portions seem larger.

44. If possible, use a teaspoon to eat or drink some of the items. Each mouthful seems to be larger.

45. If preparing a soup or casserole, do so one day ahead; refrigerate overnight. Next day, skim off fat that rises to the surface.

46. If you do use margarine or butter, let it soften to room temperature. It spreads further. Less fat and calories.

47. For a low-fat meat, try barbecuing. This process uses no butter or oils. Fat from the meat drains away during the barbecue.

48. For a low-calorie meat and poultry gravy, use bouillon. Thicken it slightly with some bran for a richer consistency.

49.   Cook brown rice or peeled, sliced potatoes in bouillon. This eliminates the need for buttering, afterwards. Serve the "natural" gravy or bouillon over the baked potatoes. Very low in calories.

50.   Whizz skim milk cottage cheese in a blender for a tasty low-calorie, low-fat substitute for sour cream.

51.   Sweeten herb tea or any beverage with a dash of cinnamon. Great for hot or cold beverages. Cinnamon eliminates the need for sugar.

52.   Add a twist of orange, lemon or lime peel to hot or iced tea for a low-calorie beverage.

53.   For a tasty "cocktail," try a glass of tomato juice with a few ice cubes and a sprinkle of lemon or lime juice.

54.   Top cooked or whole grain cereals with fresh or sun-dried fruit slices. This can replace refined sugar.

55.   Yogurt freezes well. When flavored with mashed fruit, offers a delicious alternative to ice cream! Lower in calories, too.

56.   Even if you are not on a salt fasting program, try to restrict or totally eliminate the use of this weight-causing non-food. It tends to absorb water and add weight as well as cellular bloating to the body. Restrict salt in any form and Slimfasting will be much more successful.

57.   Have someone take photographs of you from the very start of your Slimfasting and then at different stages along your program. This will give you a good Before-After image and be an incentive for you to continue.

58.   No matter what Slimfasting program you select, avoid fried foods of any sort. Reason? Whatever you fry absorbs the fat and at 225 calories per ounce of oil or grease, it gives you unwanted pounds and inches. So—bake, broil, boil, barbecue but *never* fry.

59.   Don't hold very long telephone conversations in your kitchen. It becomes tempting to snack. If this is your problem, move the phone to another part of your residence where snacking is not a temptation.

60.   Rearrange items in your refrigerator. Put foods in front that you are *least* likely to snack upon.

61.   When purchasing and preparing foods for your Slimfasting, use only the *exact* amount that you have scheduled for eating or drinking. That extra spoonful or mouthful will upset your Slimfasting program so don't have it around.

62.   Self-test yourself for those cues that may trigger off an eating urge. Whether advertisements on television, newspapers, magazines, store windows, or even menus tend to make you hungry,

avoid those circumstances during your Slimfasting—and afterwards. Avoid temptation in any form.

63. Tempted by certain very favorite foods that must be in your house for others in the family? Then make it agonizingly difficult for you to get at them. Tape shut lids of jars, cans, boxes. Make it very hard to unwrap or untie the containers and you'll feel less inclined to sneak a snack.

64. Boost your own morale with little notes and signs around the house. For example, "You'll win the battle of the bulge." Or "Get ready for a new slim shape." These give you an incentive to continue.

65. If the weather is bad, prepare for it in advance by resolving not to eat if you are confined indoors. If you cannot resist the urge to eat during "rainy day blues," then put on proper apparel and get out of the house.

You can help your body melt away those pounds and shrink those inches with dedicated Slimfasting programs and self-motivation. With these hints and tips, you can make weight losing a most rewarding experience.

HIGHLIGHTS

1. For fast weight loss, follow as many of the 65 Slimfasting hints and tips as possible.

2. Take the edge off your appetite, as did Dora MacA., with a tasty and easy-to-make *Slimfasting Tonic.*

3. A simple change in the way he ate helped Neal O'P. control his appetite. All he did was to *sit* instead of stand. This put a natural stopgap on his otherwise active appetite and he lost much weight.

4. Plan ahead for Slimfasting and use these hints and tips for greater success in swift weight loss.

Chapter Nineteen

Slimfasting Questions and Answers

Here is a roundup of questions asked by many overweights about their pounds-inches problem. By understanding the total concept of Slimfasting, you will be better able to succeed in your goal of becoming slim and trim with this technique.

"I have to attend a special affair within two weeks. My clothes are too tight. Can Slimfasting help me lose weight in time for this affair?"

You can lose more than 10 pounds if you start this Slimfasting method at once. Go on a 24 to 48 hour water fast. Then follow a selected Slimfasting program and stick to it for as close to two weeks as possible. You'll find that you'll be able to fit into your clothes and look much slimmer when you attend the special affair.

"I eat out with family and friends very often. The waiter sets very attractive (and fattening) foods before me that I feel ashamed to either avoid or restrict. What can I do?"

Begin by planning ahead. Decide you will order your own foods from the menu. Select the lowest calorie and lowest fat types of foods. You may even select a platter of raw fruits or vegetables if that is part of your current Slimfasting program. Try to select foods compatible with your program. If you are unable to eat all that is served, ask for a "doggie bag" and take the rest home. If you are sensitive about stares from others, then speak right out: "I'm on a weight losing program and can't cheat a single ounce." Don't feel embarrassed. They're *your* ugly pounds and bulgy inches and it's up to *you* to get rid of them!

"It gets to be such a bother to keep on counting calories. Must I do this all the time?"

Many of the Slimfasting programs do not call for specific calorie counts, although you'll lose more pounds and inches if you do keep a count. When Gloria J. was faced with this problem, she used a simple device: she calculated food portions in approximations of 50 and 100 calorie counts. She kept a little scorecard with the attitude that it was a daily crossword puzzle! It made calorie-carbohydrate counting a game for Gloria J. and she succeeded in losing unwanted weight.

"Much of my overeating stems from a deep-rooted nervous disorder. I do lose weight on Slimfasting but tend to fall back in my emotional disturbance and then start eating again. What can be done about this problem?"

You've taken a good step in following Slimfasting which shows you can self-motivate yourself to lose weight. To ease your nervous-emotional problems, try to get involved in a combination of physical, social and other activities. Keep your body active. Keep your mind active through *diversion, sublimation,* wherein you channel your thoughts into constructive activities. Focus attention on others and their problems. It's the best way to forget about your own. Then you'll have less of an eating urge and keep slim—while helping others.

"Much of my weight was gained after my marriage. Now the pounds and inches are stuck to me. I look at my teen-age pictures and almost weep at the way I have changed. Why is this so?"

Weight gain has nothing to do with the fact that you are married. Many folks continue eating as heavily in married life as they did when they were teen-agers. The problem is that in adulthood, a sluggish metabolism (often absent in teen-agers) causes weight build-up. Put a picture of your teen-age self on the wall. Then go on a Slimfasting program. Look at this picture often. It will motivate you to continue on the program so you can look slim again. Change your eating patterns and cut portions in half. You'll become as slim as a teen-ager if you'll eat as an adult!

"Even though my husband and I are the same age, why have I gained much more weight than he has throughout the years? I know he eats much more than I do."

After age 25, your body requires 1% less food per year because of reduced metabolic activity. By age 50, metabolism has slowed down to about 40% of what it was before. However, a woman's metabolism is even slower than that, so this is why women will often gain more weight than men even if they are the same age and even if they eat less. To correct, go on a Slimfasting program and follow the other weight control suggestions and plans in this book. If your husband is overweight, ask him to try Slimfasting. If he resists, wait until you've become slim and then he'll be convinced by proof of the pudding.

"Slimfasting helped me lose at least 9 pounds per week for close to four weeks. But the next week, all I lost were about 3 pounds. What went wrong?"

During Slimfasting, your metabolism "pulls out" fats from the fat sites in your cells, transforms them into free fatty acids, then burns them up for energy and washes out the residue. Some of the fat is also melted into a liquid which may be retained in the body for a while until it is excreted. At the start of Slimfasting, the alerted metabolism works vigorously to wash out the pounds. Later on, some of the liquefied fat tends to be retained, and this means slower weight loss. It is good to drink lots of liquids at this time to help wash out this added fat-weight. The fact that weight is being lost means Slimfasting should be continued.

"I have the urge to nibble and chew during Slimfasting. Should I try any of those sugar-free chewing gums? How about those sugar-free powdered drink mixes that put a nice flavor into water?"

Avoid any sugar-free concoctions. They have carbohydrates which add calories and upset your Slimfasting balance. They also contain synthetic chemical flavoring substances which are corrosive to your tissues and cells. To satisfy your nibbling-chewing urge, try tiny nuggets of celery, carrots, mushrooms. For beverages, try a glass of water to which you add a squeeze of lemon juice and a bit of cinnamon. Almost zero in calories and very thirst-quenching. Natural, too!

"Whenever I skip a meal or go without food, I get headaches, feel dizzy. Will this happen to me under Slimfasting?"

The circumstances are different. When you skip a meal because of pressures, it causes a headache because of the tensions involved. A pressure situation will bring on your headache and dizziness, not the food skipping. Furthermore, "unplanned for" meal skipping breaks a habit. Your subconscious and your digestion react with rebellion. This brings on the headache. But under Slimfasting, you *plan ahead* for food control. You prepare your subconscious mind, your digestion for this new change and adjustment. So there is less likelihood of any rebellious symptoms.

"During Slimfasting, is it important to select natural foods and beverages?"

Very much so. Your metabolic processes will be alerted to cleanse your cells and tissues of accumulated fats, calories and carbohydrates. It is important, therefore, to keep your system clean.

Any foods or beverages taken in should be as natural and wholesome as possible since you want to avoid cellular abuse with toxic chemicals and preservatives as found in processed items. Whether on or off Slimfasting, foods should be as natural as possible.

"Will a sauna bath, steam treatment, or massage help me lose more weight during Slimfasting?"

Heat-steam treatments help you perspire and lose much water accumulation but they may be exhausting so should be restricted in use. Massage offers some muscular vibration but does not take off pounds. If you want to keep in good physical condition, try easy walking, mild exercises as outlined in this book. Take frequent baths at home to help wash out accumulated waste-laden waters.

"Will Slimfasting help correct conditions of high blood pressure?"

High blood pressure often strikes the overweight. During Slimfasting, you will lose many pounds; this relieves the pressure of fat tightening its hold upon your viscera (internal organs) and choking off venous blood flow. Consequently, as Slimfasting takes away this fat and slims you down, there is a general loosening of the internal compression-congestion hold on your organs and there is a corresponding drop in high blood pressure. It is one of the fringe benefits of weight loss through Slimfasting.

"I love heavy, rich foods and that is why I am fat. Can Slimfasting help me, even if I have this craving for forbidden foods?"

Under a Slimfasting program, you can indulge in heavy foods that are made of polyunsaturated vegetable oils, instead of hardened fats. You can indulge in a *small portion* of your "forbidden foods" and discover it is often as satisfying as a huge amount. Under Slimfasting, try the techniques of *substitution* and *compensation*. Here's how: *substitute* skim milk cottage cheese and fresh fruit slices for an ice cream platter. *Compensate* by indulging in a thick gravy meat pie for dinner but then skip tomorrow's dinner in favor of a platter of raw fresh vegetables. This helps keep your weight in balance.

"My heavy labor job has made me bulky; while not flabby, my muscles are overweight. Can Slimfasting keep me husky but trim?"

Overweight muscles can add many unwanted pounds and inches in the wrong places. During Slimfasting on a plant food program (raw fruits, vegetables, juices, grains), your metabolism is adjusted so that energy causes capillaries to enter each muscle cell, scrub it, remove wastes and thereby help keep it slim. Slimfasting will help firm up your muscles to keep them healthy but not overburdened with fat.

"We're planning a vacation which will keep us on the beach almost all the time. We're both ashamed of our overweight figures. My husband and I want to lose unwanted weight quickly. How can we do this?"

Set your target date. Decide how many pounds you have to lose by that date. Then select a Slimfasting program immediately. You may want to start off with a 48 hour water fast. Then follow through with a day of raw fruits, then a day of raw vegetables, then a day of juices, then a day of grains. When you resume eating, do so very modestly and in smaller portions. If you stick to your schedule, you should be able to lose weight quickly, happily so you'll be slim and trim throughout your beach vacation. Finally, resolve now that you'll *remain* slim afterwards through controlled eating and regular Slimfasting.

"My wife is a terrific cook. She keeps insisting I eat and eat and eat and clean my plate. I know this is putting on more weight. How can I lose my weight but still keep my wife satisfied?"

This same problem plagued Anthony Q. who wailed that his wife was "insulted" and "hurt" if he refused to eat all she set before him. Anthony Q. solved this dilemma in a simple manner: he told his wife that she was killing him with the cruelty of enforced eating! He explained that the body requires up to ten hours to accommodate the large amount of fat-laden blood created by just one heavy meal. He explained that the liver is overburdened in its effort to metabolize the fat. Then he said that repeated heavy meals create an accumulation of supplementary fat particles in the blood which become adhered to the arteries and predispose to arteriosclerosis. So he told his wife that she could kill him with compulsory eating or extend his lifeline with moderate eating. It worked. Now Anthony Q. uses Slimfasting programs once a month and is a trim 145 pounds with a neat 34 inch waistline. His wife is convinced of his wisdom and, herself, is now svelte, thanks to Slimfasting. They eat meals regularly but not too heartily!

"For my chronic overweight, wouldn't those 'dietetic candies' do the trick?"

You're *chronically* overweight because you let your adipose cell tissues become fat and have made no effort to slim them down. So-called dietetic candies or chocolates are very high in calories. Read the label. If calories, carbohydrates, fats are *not* listed, then the manufacturer has something to hide. Pass them up. If they are listed, you'll note that just one little snack may give you 150 unwanted calories. They are of small consequence and will not do away with your appetite. They'll just tempt you to eat more of those candies and this means about 1000 extra calories with a handful of them. So . . . avoid them. They can work against you.

"When eating out, how can I follow my selected Slimfasting program?"

Very easily. As stated before, you need to plan ahead. So if you are on a raw fruit, vegetable, grain or any other type of fast, calculate how much you are scheduled to consume during mealtime and then order that particular food in the calculated amounts at the restaurant. That's all there is to it.

"Under Slimfasting, there may be a swift weight loss. Is this advisable?"

Unless you have been told otherwise, it is beneficial to lose weight rapidly to avoid the "time bomb" of ill health that may go off when you go over the limit. Slimfasting loses weight steadily, swiftly and easily so your metabolism adjusts comfortably.

"My self-motivation weakens and I feel I may not be able to continue on with Slimfasting beyond a few days. What can be done about my doubts?"

The greatest self-motivation is to see your weight dropping down. That is why you should weigh yourself daily. Here is another incentive used by Alfred C.R. Daily: He would stand completely naked before a full-length mirror, look at his heavy hanging weight, and feel ashamed of it. Then, as he saw his pounds melting on the scale, and his inches shrinking in the mirror, he developed an incentive and continued on Slimfasting. This is the simplest and often the best form of do-it-yourself behavior therapy for Slimfasting.

"On many of the Slimfasting programs, there is no need for counting calories. How can I be sure I won't take in too many calories"'

Many of the programs are planned so there is a satisfactory intake of about 1500 calories a day, even less. The permitted foods are such that they offer you appetite-digestion satisfaction with no need for counting calories. However, you should know your daily caloric need so that you don't go overboard.

"If I am on a very low calorie program, how will my body create needed energy? Many folks complain of weakness and fatigue as well as

loss of energy during a weight losing program. Is Slimfasting able to keep me energetic as pounds melt away?''

Yes. During Slimfasting, your body automatically must metabolize your stored excess fats and carbohydrates to produce energy. Slimfasting will also alert your metabolism to convert stored up protein into energy-creating carbohydrates. Generally speaking, Slimfasting enables about 10% of stored up fat and 60% of stored up protein to be transformed into energy. This gives you the vitality and vigor you need during weight loss.

"How can Slimfasting help me get rid of this bloated, heavy feeling in my stomach? (Also, I want to get rid of the bulge!)"

Slimfasting should emphasize salt-free foods so that excess water can be cast out of the system. This ends both the bloating and the bulge. Eliminate any salt-containing foods, too. This helps your body cause water loss through waste channels. This water-washing process also helps take out accumulated wastes and fats from your system.

"There are times when I feel tired or sleepy during a weight losing program. What can I do about this?"

To begin, check yourself to see if you've been getting adequate nightly sleep and make corrections. You should aim for eight hours of sound sleep. Then, if you feel afternoon fatigue, just lie down, take a nap. You'll awaken refreshed. But, if you still feel fatigued, try a glass of orange juice to which you have added a bit of honey. This alerts your metabolism, eases fatigue, gives you sparkle during Slimfasting.

"Should I try different Slimfasting programs or must I remain on just one of them at all times?"

The joy of Slimfasting is that you may go from one program to the next so that there is never any monotony or boredom. Once you have selected a program, stick to it during the time period decided upon. However, you may use one Slimfasting program at one time, then another at a different time. The point is that *you set your weight goals* and then use the Slimfasting program selected to get to your goals. You may try all-fruit, all-vegetables, all-grains, etc.

"Will I have an urge to eat after one or two days of water or liquid fasting?"

The metabolic process tends to take the edge off your appetite as fats-proteins-calories-carbohydrates *stored* in your tissues are burned up during Slimfasting. This makes you feel satisfied. But continue drinking water as much as possible so these wastes can be washed out. Water also helps keep you appetite-satisfied.

"After Slimfasting, will I have an urge to slide back to my former heavier eating ways and gain weight once again?"

Slimfasting will adjust and retrain your eating habits. Slimfasting alters and corrects your body's metabolic processes. This means you will then feel satisfied with smaller meals afterwards and will be less likely to regain unwanted pounds and inches.

"How will Slimfasting help my general health?"

Lose unwanted pounds and you gain much wanted health. If you are overweight from heavy meals, it means that your blood vessels are saturated with emulsified fat. This creates a sluggish reaction in the bloodstream. Fat particles are deposited on the inner linings of the blood vessels. There may be clogging of the choked up fatty blood channels. This may cause problems ranging from heart touble to arteriosclerosis. High fatty foods tend to cause cholesterol buildup; in many situations of arthritis, the cholesterol levels are high, which suggests that this fat is often the forerunner to this skeletal ailment. Slimfasting helps create metabolic oxidation and burning up of these fats so that you have a youthful bloodstream and healthy vessels, the very core of better health!

"I have an occasional craving for an ice cream soda. Should I indulge? I can't control myself!"

Instead of undergoing excruciating withdrawal symptoms, go ahead and have the soda. But—calculate that it will give you about 500 or more calories. Therefore, schedule a Slimfasting program that will take off 500 calories from your count.

"Is there a Slimfasting program that can give me a clean, youthful, healthy skin?"

A basic program calls for *eliminating* these foods (or items containing these foods) from your menu: oils, fats, sweets, alcohol, sugar in any form, salt in any form. Restrict them entirely. Then follow through with a raw juice fast for several days. You should be rewarded with a clean, healthy skin.

"A Slimfasting program allows me to eat 'all I want' of a few foods. Wouldn't this cause me to gain weight?"

When the program suggests "all you want" it refers to eating until your hunger is appeased. It does not mean to stuff yourself. Therefore, eat (or drink) until you're satisfied and you should lose weight since your appestat has a natural controlling device with these foods.

"My problem is that I 'eat like a bird' yet I still keep gaining weight. Why is this so? How can Slimfasting help me?"

You are nibbling constantly and this causes weight gain. Compare it to dripping faucet water in a glass. Drop by drop makes a full glass. Nibble after nibble makes pound after pound. *Total* calories and not an occasional few are what really matter. You should follow a four or five day Slimfasting program that puts you on a schedule. Retrain your appetite so you'll eat at regular times and not have to nibble.

"I have no weight problem, per se, but when I stop smoking, I have the urge to overeat. When I resume smoking, I lose weight. I want to kick the smoking habit but want to remain slim. What can I do?"

To begin with, give up smoking. Recognize that smoking usually satisfies your mouth-tongue desires. Therefore, you need to use a replacement. Try nibbling on nuggets of celery, radishes, carrots, lettuce, cucumbers. Drink lots and lots of water to wash the taste and residue of tobacco out of your system. If you are a heavy smoker, the nicotine has dulled your sense of taste so when you kick the habit, your tongue papillae become alert and now seem stronger than before. Prepare for this by satisfying your papillae with the vegetable nuggets described above. Chew, chew, chew to satisfy them further. One benefit of Slimfasting is that it helps metabolize stored up fat (often inhibited by smoking) and cast it out of the body.

"I am tapering off smoking and food at the same time. What can be done so I won't want to overeat as I kick the habit?"

DO NOT smoke either during or after a meal. Smoking will trigger off a metabolic reaction whereby there is a speedier absorption of body fat and weight gain. Set a schedule as to how few cigarettes you'll smoke daily. Each day, smoke one or two fewer cigarettes. Smoke them *between* meals so they don't interfere with your Slimfasting metabolic processes. Gradually, as you lower cigarette intake, you'll be able to get rid of the smoking urge and overeating urge, too.

With Slimfasting, your lean-trim future is in your hands—and mouth, too! It's easy to lose unwanted pounds and inches with your hands and mouth. Your reward will be a youthful body and mind. It is your pot of gold at the end of the Slimfasting rainbow.

SUMMARY

1. Erase doubts about Slimfasting by noting the answers to many common and uncommon questions about weight losing.

2. Gloria J. took the confusion out of calorie counting. She pre-calculated most food portions in approximations of 50 and 100 calorie counts. A scorecard told her how many calories she was taking daily through selected food portions.

3. Anthony Q. pleased his wife who ordinarily felt hurt if he refused her overabundant supplies of food with a simple explanation. Now, both have re-trained their eating habits and are slimmer (and healthier, too!) because of it.

4. Alfred C.R. used a simple and totally free self-motivational step that made him eager to continue with Slimfasting. It was the greatest incentive he needed.

Chapter Twenty

How to Be "Forever Slim"
and Youthful
with Lifetime Slimfasting

To be "forever slim" and "fat free" it is important to plan for frequent Slimfasting programs. Once you have scheduled your Slimfasting, you can look forward to being youthfully trim without the problem of burdensome pounds and bulging inches. Here is a round-up of some of the best benefits that await you on a Slimfasting program.

SLIMFASTING MELTS AWAY OVERWEIGHT
IN A SHORT TIME

Once you follow a scheduled Slimfasting program and have set your goals, your alerted metabolism will "trigger" off your body's built-in pound-melting process. This process alerts your entire body and creates a calorie-carbohydrate-fat melting response that can take pounds off at the rate of one to two pounds a day. Inches go down as much as one inch per day. Slimfasting also works overnight, while you sleep. In effect, you go to sleep overweight and wake up much slimmer.

SLIMFASTING SEPARATES HUNGER
FROM APPETITE   .

Much overweight is traced to an insatiable or uncontrollable hunger urge. During Slimfasting, there is a readjustment of your body's appetite mechanism so that hunger will just about abate. Your mouth and tongue become re-educated as they are cleansed of toxins. You develop a healthy sense of taste and a natural appetite so that you will later eat until nutritionally satisified and feel comfortable even with moderate portions. Slimfasting trains you so that you will then have a healthy appetite without the temptation to overeat.

SLIMFASTING ADJUSTS
YOUR METABOLIC CLOCKS

The key to weight loss is in a healthy metabolism that burns up excess fat-causing elements. Healthy food is needed to nourish your digestive system, to alert your glands and help adjust the rhythm of your metabolic clock system. Slimfasting tends to adjust these metabolic clocks within your system. As a result, Slimfasting corrects the metabolic clock so that endocrine adjustments make food assimilation more efficient. Slimfasting corrects the basic problem wherein an erroneous metabolism converts glucose to fat much too rapidly and does not produce sufficient energy. This re-direction of the endocrine secretions so that glucose can be used for energy with less fat conversion means there is less weight gain. Slimfasting is able to adjust this metabolic mechanism within your system.

SLIMFASTING CREATES A FEELING
OF REJUVENATION

When the toxic wastes are washed out of your system, when your viscera and the billions of body cells and tissues are washed of their accumulated weighty substances, there is a total feeling of youthful health. There is a corresponding resurgence of youthful vitality. Many folks say they feel improved breathing, freedom from aches and arthritic-like pains, clearer skin, clearer eyesight, and even better hearing. The correction of body chemistry creates improvement in the taste buds so that there is a natural craving for more healthful foods. It is a total remaking of the entire body and mind, too. This creates a feeling of overall rejuvenation.

SLIMFASTING CLEANSES INTERNAL ORGANS

During Simfasting, your body starts to draw upon its accumulated reserves and stored up substances. It draws on fat, cells, tissues, muscles, blood, water. It is a form of internal self-cleansing. In the absence of burdensome food, the metabolic process now must turn inward for sustenance and this creates a self-cleansing reaction. At the end of Slimfasting, the cleansed organs are now ready to function at efficient speed and youthful vitality through this washing action.

SLIMFASTING IMPROVES EMOTIONAL HEALTH

Basically, your central nervous system requires blood sugar (glucose) for nourishment. This glucose is made available by carbohydrates from foods. During Slimfasting, the body's own built-in storage system sends a supply of needed glucose to the central nervous system so it can function healthfully. Without the burden of accumulating food, the nervous system can now be nourished by glucose and help improve emotional health.

Your brain, too, requires glucose daily in the amounts of about 125 grams. During Slimfasting, some glucose is taken from the liver's reserve of glycogen and then from protein. Liver-stored glucose is comparable to food glucose, which is needed to energize the brain and provide you with youthful thinking powers. During Slimfasting, this supply is made more readily available. Furthermore, the brain swiftly adapts ketones as a substitute source of emotional energy so you will be rewarded with emotional and mental vitality during Slimfasting.

SLIMFASTING: THE ALL-PURPOSE
INTERNAL CLEANSER

Slimfasting creates this all-purpose internal cleansing action: Energy that is ordinarily devoted to assimilation is now spared the labor of food digestion. It is now used to expel the accumulation of waste matter and weight-causing debris that clings to the cells and organs. Slimfasting also helps cleanse the alimentary canal of potentially harmful bacteria and wastes. (This canal consists of the entire digestive tract: mouth, pharynx, esophagus, stomach and intestine.) Once these are eliminated, healthy vitamins may be synthesized in the intestine for better digestion. You will experience a coated tongue, unpleasant breath, debris-laden mouth. This is the reaction of Slimfasting since wastes are coming up, toxic substances including food additives and air pollutants are being removed from your body. Slimfasting also creates a toxin-flushing response wherein the digestive tract is ridding your body of the keto acids in the blood. These wastes need to be detoxified and eliminated from the system. It is part of the "total rejuvenation" process of weight-losing Slimfasting.

TWELVE BASIC SLIMFASTING RULES

1. *Before You Begin:* Prepare yourself emotionally for Slimfasting, at least two or three days before. Skip an occasional meal in

advance so your system will slowly adjust to the program. Be sure to drink lots of water. Also increase your intake of fresh fruits and vegetables about three days before your Slimfasting. This is important. This will help give you needed bulk and roughage to promote regularity. You should also increase intake of whole grains such as bran to further create regularity.

2. *Drink Two Quarts of Water Daily During Slimfasting.* It helps wash out accumulated debris from your system. It also helps keep you filled up and satisfied. Plan to drink at least two quarts of water daily.

3. *Get a Good Night's Sleep.* Each and every night of Slimfasting calls for sound sleep. You'll note that the diuretic (water loss) reaction of Slimfasting will also make you feel calm and rested so that sleep will come easily. But you should rest nightly with refreshing sleep.

4. *Keep Active within Reason.* Physical activity helps alert your various systems. Walking, mild games are helpful. But guard against too vigorous activities. As your body is undergoing adjustments, you may become dizzy if you make swift, jerky movements. So keep active within moderate reason.

5. *Keep Your Body Warm.* Avoid chills, drafts. Avoid sudden temperature changes such as going from an air-conditioned room into the hot outdoors. Give yourself a little time in a vestibule to make adjustments. Keep your hands and feet warm. If it is chilly at night, use a blanket.

6. *Bathe Yourself in Tepid Water.* Bath or shower water should be tepid. Do not take any hot baths. They can be enervating and upset your metabolism.

7. *Avoid Sudden, Abrupt Motions.* Do not jump out of a chair too rapidly. Do not leap out of bed with a jerky motion. Do not bend over too swiftly or without some preparation. You should do everything with casual, gentle motions. Your head may spin, otherwise, because of abrupt motions.

8. *Medications, Drugs, Pills on Doctor's Advice Only.* During Slimfasting, the reduction in food will make your organs more delicate and medication may be harsh. So any of these drugs should be taken with your doctor's advice only. Tell him you are fasting so he will understand your situation.

9. *Do Not Smoke.* If you have a smoking habit, prepare to give it up during Slimfasting. It is upsetting and poisonous to introduce nicotine and other chemicals into a fasting organism (and under other conditions, too!). You'll find that Slimfasting will help you kick the smoking habit.

10. *Do Not Drink Alcohol.* You'll be "scorching" your liver and upsetting your metabolism with any alcoholic beverages. Again, Slimfasting will help you resist the drinking urge and you'll probably be able to kick this habit, too.

11. *Use Natural Dentifrice.* Commercial toothpaste, tooth powder, and mouthwashes contain artificial ingredients and corrosive chemicals so avoid their use. To keep your mouth and teeth and tongue clean, use a little baking soda in a glass of warm water as a wash. Brush teeth and scrub tongue with a bit of baking soda.

12. *Break Your Fast with Preparation and Slowness.* A day before your scheduled ending, prepare yourself to break the fast. Do so gradually on the selected day. Food and beverage intake should be very slight. Eat very slowly. Do not suddenly overburden your resting digestive system. If you stuff yourself you may feel nausea. Avoid salt and harsh seasonings since these may cause edema (cellular swelling of the tissues). Gradually resume more healthful eating patterns.

You'll discover that not only do you emerge from Slimfasting with lost weight but with better health. You'll also find that food is no longer such a temptation as before. You'll enjoy more healthful foods and in reasonable quantities so the threat of overweight is as reduced as your body weight!

BASIC SLIMFASTING PROGRAM

Vivian V. had a weight problem that made her bulge in all the wrong places. But as an active housewife, she is always tasting and nibbling foods that she is preparing. This adds on unwanted weight. So she follows a simple basic Slimfasting program whenever she notices her scales show she has gained ten pounds over her desired weight. Here is the program that keeps Vivian V. slim and trim within her weight goals:

FIRST DAY. Drink nothing but water. Eat absolutely nothing.

SECOND DAY. Drink just one glass of fruit juice. Drink as much water as is desired throughout the day.

THIRD DAY. Drink just one glass of vegetable juice. Drink as much water as is desired throughout the day.

FOURTH DAY. Drink one glass of fruit juice. Drink one glass of vegetable juice. Drink as much water as is desired throughout the day.

FIFTH DAY. Take the first solid food in the form of well-chewed fruits in moderation. Drink one glass of fruit juice. Drink one glass of vegetable juice. Drink as much water as is desired throughout the day.

SIXTH DAY. Take more solid food. Space intake of well-chewed fruits and vegetables. Drink one glass of fruit juice. Drink one glass of vegetable juice. Drink as much water as is desired throughout the day.

SEVENTH DAY. Start to ease out of the Slimfasting with more well-chewed fruits and vegetables, cooked whole grains, several glasses of fruit and vegetable juice.

POUNDS, INCHES MELT AWAY

This easy seven day Slimfasting program has helped Vivian V. maintain her slim 112 pound weight level so that she need not worry about gaining too much. It's the easy and (important to her) swift way to lose weight. She finds that this basic and simple Slimfasting program keeps weight off so that if she does not snack or nibble, she is *permanently slim!*

Establish Weight Limit—Schedule Slimfasting

To enjoy the benefits of being "forever slim," just follow this simple two step program: (1) Establish your weight limit. Decide how much you should weigh. Then decide that if you go five or more pounds above that limit, you need to Slimfast. (2) Schedule Slimfasting as soon as you see that you have gone over the weight limit. This will help keep you slim.

Correct Basic Eating Practices

Slimfasting will help readjust your metabolic processes so that you will have a lessened desire for overeating. But you should correct your basic eating practices to avoid poisoning your system.

As stated throughout this book, your eating practices should emphasize wholesome, natural foods. Avoid salt and sugar in any form. Avoid tobacco and alcohol in any form. Avoid fried foods in any form. You will thereby be nourishing and healing your body with good foods. These antagonists are to be avoided since they abuse your body.

GIVE UP JUNK FOOD

This is not deprivation. It is good health. Your billions of body cells and tissues are created to give you good health. This is possible through self-regeneration of Slimfasting and the introduction of healthy and not abusive junk food. Basically, remove the cause of overweight: namely being overburdened with toxins as found in processed, refined and chemicalized foods. Unhealthy food can cause unhealthy weight gain. Once Slimfasting has washed out the debris, change your eating practices to include natural and wholesome foods.

SLIMFASTING CORRECTS EATING URGE

Once the autolysis or self-digesting action of Slimfasting has scrubbed and washed your viscera and cells of weighty-wastes, you will notice a correction in your eating urge. There is a difference between appetite and hunger. *Appetite* is the urge to stuff yourself to fill a deep-seated emotional need. *Hunger* is the instinctive requirement to give good nourishment to your body. Slimfasting resets your metabolic clocks so that your appetite is controlled and hunger now takes the scene and you will eat for nourishment and not emotional upset.

Basically, Slimfasting enables every single segment of your body to transform into low gear; then, the body can shed weight, toxic wastes (blocked energy) and debris. It is the simple way to rejuvenated health.

Select your desired type of Slimfasting according to taste and variety and enjoy this ancient method for weight loss and youthful health.

Once your body has switched over to fat metabolism, once the cleansing process has taken hold, once the pounds and inches leave your body, you will be experiencing a complete revitalization from head to toe.

When you resume your regular eating patterns after Slimfasting, select healthy and wholesome foods. You will then be able to remain slim, maintain a high energy state, and feel youthful because of better assimilation of food by a rested and burden-free system.

Slimfasting is an ancient secret of swift weight loss. You can use this secret in our modern times and tap the wells of health within your own body to experience rebirth and regeneration with weight loss. Today may well be the first day of the rest of your slim life!

SUMMARY

1. Slimfasting retrains your physical and emotional eating habits and builds a "forever slim" longer lifespan.
2. Note the 12 basic Slimfasting rules for before, during and after.
3. Follow the Basic Slimfasting Program as does Vivian V. for lifetime slimness and good health.

Weight Problem Solvamatic Index